ABOUT THE AUTHOR

Lesley Reynolds has been at the forefront of skincare for more than twenty years and there isn't anything she doesn't know about the world of anti-ageing, aesthetic treatments and skincare. She currently runs a successful clinic on London's Harley Street with her husband, where they offer cutting-edge treatments as well as anti-ageing advice to media and celebrity clients.

To my wonderful Father and Mother and family who have given me so much love, support and laughter and put up with my antisocial hours whilst writing this book. I love you all.

EASY WAYS TO DROP A DECADE

Secrets From Harley Street

Lesley Reynolds

MACMILLAN

This edition first published 2012 by Macmillan
Previously published 2010 as *Look Younger for Longer* by Rodale
Imprints of Pan Macmillan Ltd
Pan Macmillan, 20 New Wharf Road, London N1 9RR
Basingstoke and Oxford
Associated companies throughout the world
www.panmacmillan.com

ISBN 978-0-230-76921-2

3 5 7 9 8 6 4 2

A CIP catalogue record for this book is available from the British Library.

Text designed by seagulls.net

Printed and bound by CPI Group (UK) Ltd, Croydon, CR0 4YY

This book is intended as a reference volume only, not as a medical manual. The information given here is designed to help you make informed decisions about your health. It is not intended as a substitute for any treatment that you may have been prescribed by your doctor. If you suspect you have a medical problem, we urge you to seek competent medical help.

Mention of specific companies, organizations or authorities in this book does not imply endorsement by the publisher, nor does mention of specific companies, organizations or authorities in the book imply that they endorse the book.

Addresses, websites and telephone numbers given in this book were correct at the time of going to press.

Visit **www.panmacmillan.com** to read more about all our books and to buy them. You will also find features, author interviews and news of any author events, and you can sign up for e-newsletters so that you're always first to hear about our new releases.

Contents

Introduction

I've spent more than 20 years in the beauty business, helping women from all walks of life to look younger for longer. Running a busy skincare clinic on London's Harley Street means I speak to thousands of women every year about their looks. Each one comes in for a different reason, but the one thing they all have in common is the desire to look their absolute best for as long as possible.

The great news is that these days we have many wonderful anti-ageing tools available to us. I can honestly say there has never been a more exciting time in anti-ageing, which is why I was passionate about writing this book. I felt it was the perfect time to share all my insider secrets to looking younger, the treatments my celebrity clients swear by and the products I know will help you achieve glowing, radiant skin.

My aim is to cut through many of the beauty myths out there and guide you step-by-step through my tried-and-tested methods to maintain, improve and care for your skin from top to toe. I'll share all my best tips for every part of the body, from DIY fixes that anyone can try, to non-invasive clinic treatments and injectables, and finally, as a last resort, surgical procedures.

In my mother's day, anti-ageing didn't involve much more than applying a generous helping of cold cream, crossing your fingers and hoping Mother Nature would be kind to you as the years went by. Today, though, things couldn't be more different. Ingredients that used to be confined to high-end products in clinics have made their way into high-street creams, and non-surgical procedures such as fillers, peels or Botox, which only a few years ago used to be the preserve of wealthy women or Hollywood A-listers, now don't cost the earth.

But with so many anti-ageing products and treatments on the market, it can be a minefield out there when it comes to working out which ones are best for you.

I've had many clients who've spent hundreds of pounds on creams, purchased because they were a 'beauty editor's favourite' in a glossy magazine, which now sit on the bathroom shelf only half-used because they haven't fulfilled their expectations. Have you ever noticed how many of the products that come highly recommended or win awards in women's magazines are the ones that have bought advertising space in the very same issues? Worth thinking about...

I've devoted a whole chapter to de-jargoning these lotions and potions (see Chapter 5), revealing the best ingredients to look for in anti-ageing products and giving you my expert opinion on the results you can realistically expect to get from them.

I'm often frustrated by the messages sent out to women by the beauty industry. Adverts for anti-ageing products that use gorgeous models in their 20s with flawless, airbrushed skin create an image that's unachievable for the majority of us and just leave us with a sinking feeling, particularly when we look in the mirror and are treated to the sight of puffy eyes or a droopy jowl. It's not a positive message, not least because if you're reading this (and buying anti-ageing products) you've probably said goodbye to your 20s a few years ago. I strongly believe that the key to anti-ageing is to look the very best you can for your age – whatever that is.

Through running my clinic, I've been lucky to gain an insight into how real women think and feel about the ageing process and for me there's nothing more satisfying than seeing the transformation that simply using the right skincare can have, not only on a woman's complexion, but also on her self-confidence. I hope the advice in this book will bring out the best in you, too.

One of the most exciting areas in anti-ageing in recent years has been non-surgical treatments such as lasers and injectables and, throughout the book, I've talked about the best ones to target individual age-related problems. More often than not these treatments are a more effective (and much cheaper) alternative to going under the knife. And, unlike surgery, there's little or no downtime and a minimal risk of scarring. I've road-tested many of the treatments mentioned in this book – peels, fillers, laser resurfacing, Botox – so I can tell you the honest truth about the results, as well as the ouch factor!

A good cosmetic doctor will always take a subtle approach to anti-ageing. These days it's all about using a combination of non-surgical options and making small tweaks over time to achieve a natural result that helps you look fabulous for the age that you are. We've all seen those women who've had 'too much work' and I think you'll agree that it doesn't make them look younger; it just makes them look different. It's far better to look fabulous for 45 rather than a ropey 38-year-old!

Face-lifts were once the only option if you wanted to hold back the years, but they are now seen as old-fashioned because of the big advances in non-surgical treatments. I'd never recommend surgery as a first-line treatment, but I have mentioned a few 'nip tuck' options at the end of each chapter because there are problems, such as a bad case of turkey neck or fat that slides down to form ridges under the eyes, that no exercise, cream, laser or injectable will shift. So it's useful to know what the options are and what you can expect.

It's also important to remember that your body changes with the passage of time and what looked good at 40 might look very strange at 70. This is why you should think long and hard about having a surgical procedure that alters your face or body permanently. I'll never forget a gorgeous old lady in her 70s, who came to see me about a dry skin problem. When she disrobed I was confronted with what I can only describe as two Madeleine cakes for breasts! She had an incredibly pert bosom, which frankly looked wrong and pretty shocking for a woman of her age. I decided there and then never to go too far with any type of cosmetic procedure.

Before they even start thinking about getting rid of their lines, I always advise clients to look at improving their skin first. In our clinic we always start by working on the condition of clients' skin – tackling open pores, banishing blemishes, improving skin texture and repairing sun damage. That's why there's a whole chapter (see Chapter 2) dedicated to good skincare habits and simply treating your face and body with tender loving care to achieve fresher, smoother, more radiant skin. How you treat your skin on a daily basis can make a huge difference to its quality and affect how well it ages.

There is a huge amount you can do yourself when it comes to looking younger for longer, so this book is packed with DIY tips and natural helpers to tackle every part of your body – from eye bags to wobbly thighs.

I believe one of the most important things any woman can do as the years go by is to evolve her look. Anti-ageing isn't about desperately trying to appear 20-something for ever; that way lies the slippery slope into mutton dressed as lamb territory. It's about looking fabulous for the age that you are and feeling comfortable in your own skin. There are many simple ways to update your look which won't blow the budget or require an appointment with a cosmetic doctor, and you'll find them all in Chapter 4. This chapter is a goldmine of brilliant fashion, hair and make-up tricks and if you use them, you'll leave people astonished when you reveal your real age.

Staying youthful is a lot about attitude, too. The best thing about getting older is that you have more confidence in yourself and have learned over the years what suits you. So harness this and make it work for you. There's nothing more attractive than a woman who is confident in who she is.

In fact, I believe looking your best is a lot to do with how you feel on the inside. For me, the people who look old before they should are the ones who are stressed and miserable. It's amazing how a smile lifts your entire face. Happiness also boosts those all-important feelgood hormones, giving you a radiant glow that no miracle cream will be able to recreate. So it's important for all of us to work on wellbeing, and try to find a balance in our super-busy and demanding twenty-first-century lives. That means managing stress better, taking care of our diet, staying active, getting our beauty sleep – basically nourishing our skin from the inside. Easier said than done, right? Well, Chapter 3 is packed to the brim with lifestyle advice to help you do all of those things.

I wholeheartedly believe the best way to tackle ageing is with a holistic approach – good lifestyle habits and products combined with the best treatments salons and clinics have to offer. And I hope this book will give you all the tools and information you need to do just that.

Unlike our mothers, we're lucky to live in a period when greater knowledge and state-of-the-art skin treatments mean it's never been easier to hold back the years and remain youthful and vital as the decades pass. I hope you'll be inspired by the book to believe that you, too, can embrace and enjoy those advancing years, confident that there's so much you can do to stay looking fabulous.

So raise your glasses, ladies, and make a toast to looking younger for longer!

Lesley x

TIP! You'll find stockists for all the products listed in the book, along with some useful websites, on page 277.

one

Your Face and Body Through the Decades

Let's face it – nobody enjoys the effect growing older has on our looks, and anyone who says differently is lying. Sadly, there is no 'Peter Pan' miracle that can stop your body clock as the decades pass; ageing is as inevitable as the changing seasons.

On the other hand, there are lots of things you can do to wrestle back some power from Father Time and ensure you look younger for longer. Picking up healthy habits – such as wearing sunscreen every day – can go a long way towards preserving that fresh bloom of youth.

We all have a favourite time of life when we feel and look our absolute best, and many of you reading this book still have that to come! For lots of women this isn't the 20s, as you might expect. You may have been slim and wrinkle-free at 21 but you didn't have the confidence to enjoy it or hadn't learnt how to make the most of your looks, so you would therefore pick a later decade as your beauty peak.

Personally, I think many women look their most gorgeous at the happiest times in their lives: when they fall in love, during their first years of marriage, after getting their dream job, when their kids go to school or leave home and they have more time to themselves.

My magic age was 38. I loved it. I adored my hair, felt good about my body, I had bags of self-confidence, and had only just started getting a few lines – just enough to give my face a bit of character. But even though I'm now 20 years older, I'm probably happier than ever before and I wouldn't turn back the clock. I have three gorgeous children, a great husband, a fabulous job and a wonderful family around me. My skin is a lot crinklier, but five out of six isn't bad!

The ageing process is swings and roundabouts, bringing extra wrinkles along with wisdom, confidence and peace of mind. As the still-fabulous 50-something actress Michelle Pfeiffer said: 'If you think hitting 40 is liberating, just wait till you hit 50.'

For me, the key to feeling beautiful through every decade is accepting your reflection. Too often women hold on to a self-image from a time that's long gone. This younger self is how we secretly hope we'll always appear, so it can be a nasty shock to catch sight of yourself in a shop window and find the woman looking back at you isn't a fresh-faced ingénue. If this sounds at all familiar, you need to make the mirror your friend, not your enemy. Accept that both your face and your body are going to change over time, then focus on making the most of how you look in each decade.

Think of your 18-year-old self as an old friend, and accept that while her beauty regime may have brought out the best in her, it won't do the same for you. Your regime must adapt and evolve as you do. Don't be surprised when the miracle moisturiser you've loved for the past ten years stops working, or your old diet rules such as 'only eat dessert every other day' are no longer keeping you slim.

As we get older our requirements change, and each decade needs a fresh approach to make-up, skincare, diet and exercise to keep us looking fabulous.

In this chapter, I'll give you a snapshot of what each decade has in store for your face and body, and reveal how to adapt your beauty and lifestyle habits accordingly. But first, let's talk about the factors that influence how we age.

How your skin ages

The most noticeable signs of ageing are the changes that occur in your facial skin – yes, we're talking wrinkles, age spots, sagging and dryness. Sadly, we're all familiar with these ageing giveaways, but what is actually happening to your skin to make these signs appear?

Your skin consists of two layers: the epidermis (outer) and the dermis (inner). The cells that make up the epidermis on your skin's surface are continuously shed and replaced by newer cells from deeper layers of the epidermis. This process, known as skin renewal, keeps your skin looking fresh. The dermis underneath is basically a network of collagen and elastin fibres that provide your skin with support, elasticity and that youthful plumpness.

From your late 20s, your rate of skin renewal starts to slow down. As this happens, the surface of your skin becomes thinner, making it more prone to environmental damage from the sun, cold weather and pollution. A build-up of dead skin cells also causes your complexion to look duller and more uneven.

At the same time, the collagen and elastin fibres deeper down in your skin begin to break down and your ability to produce more fibres starts to slow. This is what causes fine lines, wrinkles, and loose, sagging skin.

Finally, your skin generally becomes drier with age, as the lipids – a waxy substance that creates a barrier against water loss – start to break down as a result of changes in hormone levels due to the menopause. This means the barrier becomes leaky, allowing more water to escape from the skin, causing dehydration and flakiness.

The age factor

How well or how much we age is never down to just one factor; there is always a combination of genetic and lifestyle influences at play. And although some factors, such as our mother's tendency to eye bags, might be beyond our control, others, including sun protection and using the right beauty products, can be harnessed and used in the battle against ageing through every decade.

Here are the main factors that affect how our skin ages.

ALL IN THE GENES?

Have you ever wondered why some people look as though they're in their 20s when they're actually closer to 40? The answer usually lies in their genes. Just as the genetic blueprint we inherit from our parents determines our hair and eye colour, it also plays a big part in how we age.

If you want a good indicator of how your skin and body are going to change as you grow older just take a look at your parents and grandparents. One US skin study found that mothers and daughters aged in remarkably similar ways, even down to the exact age at which tell-tale signs such as laughter lines started to appear.

Your genes control several natural processes that cause your skin to age, and it appears that some people are simply genetically programmed to age more slowly when it comes to skin texture, tone, and elasticity.

However, if you fear turning into a carbon copy of your mother you should take heart from the fact that many other signs of ageing – such as fine lines around the mouth and age spots – are strongly influenced by environmental factors, which can be avoided.

AMOUNT OF SUN EXPOSURE

The single biggest cause of premature skin ageing is repeated, long-term exposure to the sun. Dermatologists call this kind of skin damage 'photo-ageing', and it's caused by the sun's ultraviolet rays.

Ultraviolet (UV) light causes the skin to produce too much pigment, which results in the formation of freckles and age spots. UV light also accelerates the breakdown of those all-important collagen and elastin fibres, which causes the skin to sag, wrinkle and become rough and leathery. When it's sun-damaged skin also bruises and tears more easily, and takes longer to heal.

Unsurprisingly, people who spend a significant amount of time outdoors without proper protection experience deeper lines and wrinkles and greater skin sagging than those who are careful to avoid sun damage. Even more seriously, UV light can damage the DNA in skin cells, which can lead to different forms of skin cancer.

Most women love to get a bit a sun on their face, blissfully unaware that the signs of photo-ageing can lie invisible beneath the surface of their skin for years. As a result, they might become complacent or even

TIP! Sunshine on our skin creates vitamin D, which we need for good health. If you have fair skin you'll need between five and ten minutes of unprotected sun exposure on your arms and legs three times a week. If you have a medium skin tone, you'll need between 15 and 20 minutes and dark skins may need up to 30 minutes. Most of us get enough exposure just going about our everyday lives – walking to work or the shops, taking the dog for a walk and so on. Whenever you're in daylight you're getting exposure to UV rays, even through windows.

addicted to sunbathing – but just a few minutes of sun exposure each day is enough to cause noticeable changes in the skin over the years.

The good news is that this is one form of ageing you can prevent. The simple answer is to wear a suncream containing an SPF (sun protection factor) of at least 15 – whatever the weather or season, as UV rays can still cause damage even on cloudy winter days. SPF 15 is the minimum strength but, for real protection from the ageing effects of the sun, I'd always recommend SPF 30 in the summer months.

SMOKING

If you want to stay youthful, a zero-tolerance approach to smoking is your only option. After UV damage, smoking is one of the main environmental factors that causes premature ageing in women. Smoke affects the flexibility of skin leading to wrinkles and a leathery texture – and the damage it does inside is even worse.

Smoking activates the genes responsible for a skin enzyme that breaks down existing collagen in the skin, and also slows down the production of new collagen, causing your skin to lose its elasticity, leading to sagging and wrinkles.

The nicotine in cigarettes causes the tiny blood vessels in your skin to become narrower. This lessens the blood flow to your skin, depriving it of oxygen and important nutrients, such as vitamin A – yet another cause of premature ageing.

Cigarettes rob your skin of vitamin C, and no matter how much you take as a supplement, you just can't absorb enough to replenish what is lost.

If all that wasn't enough, repeated exposure to the heat from burning cigarettes and the facial expressions you make while smoking – such as pursing your lips and squinting your eyes – all contribute to wrinkles. Just look at the face of a lifelong smoker to see what I mean.

The best beauty treatment for smokers by far is simply to quit. The ageing effects of cigarettes can be greatly diminished, and in some cases completely avoided, if you give up. Even people who have smoked for many years, or who smoked heavily at a younger age, show less facial wrinkling and improved skin tone once they quit.

However, the sooner you kick the habit the better as far as your skin is concerned. One recent study found that facial wrinkling, while not yet visible, could be seen under a microscope in smokers as young as 20!

DIET

When it comes to food, I'm afraid we still haven't found the perfect elixir of youth. Nevertheless, what you drink and eat over the years does have a profound effect on how your skin ages. Alcohol is dehydrating and dilates blood vessels, which can show up as spider veins on your face. Meanwhile, foods rich in natural age-fighting vitamins called antioxidants, such as brightly coloured fruit and veg, can play their part in fresher, healthier skin. In other words, if you eat a healthy, balanced diet you're already doing a fair bit to ward off premature ageing. For advice on foods with the best beauty benefits, see pages 58–65.

Keeping a steady weight is your best bet when it comes to looking youthful, as years of ballooning followed by sudden weight loss when you diet can take its toll on your face. I talk more about yo-yo dieting on page 66 as I feel strongly about it; some women put themselves through these cycles for many years without realising the long-term effects they can have on their health as well as their looks.

STRESS LEVELS

Have you ever noticed how facial expressions are different when some-one is under stress? Their brow furrows and forms a deep frown line – a real age giveaway. Meanwhile, a person who is stress-free and happy can appear years younger, as their facial muscles are more relaxed.

Recently experts have been paying more attention to the connection between the brain and the skin, an area they call 'psychodermatology'. Studies show that stressful emotions can unleash a torrent of stress hormones, such as cortisol, which cause blood vessels to constrict, reducing the amount of essential nutrients our skin receives. This process not only ages our skin, but can also trigger a wide range of allergic and inflammatory skin ailments.

Stressed-out people suffer from lower levels of the anti-stress hormone DHEA (dehydroepiandrosterone), which has been shown in numerous studies to help maintain the youthfulness of skin cells.

The meaning of all this complicated science is actually very simple: reducing the level of stress in your life will keep your skin looking younger for longer.

There's no point investing in fancy moisturisers if you don't also take the time to work out what factors cause the most hassle in your life. And while it's obviously not possible to eliminate all your stress triggers – unless you completely ignore your husband and kids and give up work for good – you can still strive to find better ways to cope with some of them. (See Chapter 3, page 57 for some ideas.)

YOUR SKIN TYPE

Different skin types age differently, so identifying what type you have will help you understand how it will age and ensure you use the right prod-ucts to control it.

There are four main skin types:

- Despite the name, 'normal' skin is very rare in adults. It's similar to baby skin and has a uniform texture with small or invisible pores and no blackheads. Normal skin is soft and does not feel tight after cleansing. If well looked after, it won't wrinkle until later in life.
- Oily skin is thicker than other skin types, and normally feels greasy and shiny. The pores are bigger and prone to spots and blackheads. But on the plus side, oily skin ages better than other types because the oily coating makes it more resistant to external factors such as sun damage.
- Dry skin produces less sebum and has difficulty retaining moisture, so it often has a dull appearance and can feel tight, or flaky. Expression lines form faster in dry skin, especially around the eyes and mouth, and it can develop a sallow tone.
- Combination skin is oily around the T-zone (forehead, nose and chin) and normal or dry over the rest of the face. As a result it can age faster around the drier areas such as the cheeks and eyes.

If you're not sure which type of skin you have, try this little test to find out. First, cleanse your face with a wash-off cleanser, then wait for an hour. Once the time is up, press a tissue to your face and look at it for the following signs:

- If your skin is normal, you'll see nothing on the tissue and it will slide off your skin like silk.
- If your skin is combination, you'll see an imprint of oil from the T-zone areas.
- If it's dry, you'll feel flaky, rough skin rubbing on the tissue and your skin will probably feel quite tight, too.
- If it's oily skin you have, the tissue will have oil all over it.

TIP! These days, many people have sensitivities brought on by a reaction to certain chemical ingredients in skincare products (see page 36 for information on the common culprits). If this is the case for you, choose simple products with few ingredients, and go for natural and organic ranges to avoid flare-ups.

When it comes to an anti-ageing beauty routine, sadly there's no one-size-fits-all regime that works for everyone. This means you're going to have to try out a few different creams and brands before finding the ones that suit you.

The single most important product in your fight against premature ageing is, of course, your moisturiser. When skin is dry, the cells become shrivelled, creating fine lines and wrinkles long before they're due. So although moisturisers can't actually prevent wrinkles forming – whatever the packaging may claim – they will hydrate your skin, plumping it up and improving its overall appearance.

When it comes to anti-ageing products, it's important to note that the price of an anti-ageing skincare cream is not an accurate indication of its effectiveness. Numerous studies from around the world have shown that there is often not much difference in the results produced by the most expensive anti-ageing creams and the bargain basement ones.

The only thing that matters when it comes to wrinkle-fighting is the active ingredients a product contains. As a rule of thumb, if your cream doesn't contain ingredients proven to work, such as retinol or alpha hydroxy acids (AHAs), then it won't do anything more than hydrate your skin. So always do some research and check the label before you part with your cash. (See pages 110–30 for my expert guide to choosing the right anti-ageing products from the hundreds out there.)

In my experience, following the right rules can dramatically slow down the ageing process. Combining the correct skincare products and lifestyle choices can give you good deal of control over how youthful you look, but the needs of your skin change as you get older. A 50-year-old needs a different regime to a 20-year-old. Before we go any further, here is my easy-to-follow, top-to-toe guide for every age, decade by decade.

Your 20s

If you're still in your 20s, be sure to appreciate what you have, because as the decades go by, you're going to have to work harder and harder at looking good. Efforts put in now to protect your skin will pay dividends in later decades and you'll be very glad you bothered.

SKIN

During this decade of youthful promise your skin is still blissfully wrinkle-free and glowing – so be sure to enjoy it! Your skin cells are renewing monthly and collagen levels are at an all-time high, making it the perfect time to capitalise on the fact that everything's working in your favour. But don't be fooled into thinking your skin will be fresh forever, or can recover from whatever toxins you throw at it during your party decade. Before your 20s are out, your cell turnover rate will be starting to slow and it won't be long before you notice a slight loss of freshness and firmness, so now's the time to get into the habit of exfoliating your face and body a couple of times a week. Establishing a thorough skincare routine now will help you to keep looking this good for as long as possible.

Skin savers

- If you invest in just one beauty product, make it sun protection – it's the absolute best (and cheapest) way to ensure your youthful looks last. Wear a really good sunscreen, with an SPF of at least 15, every day of the year.
- If you're comfortable doing so, go without make-up entirely to let your skin breathe and just slather on a good SPF moisturiser to let your natural glow shine through. Alternatively, apply a light dusting of mineral make-up, which won't clog your pores.
- You can be prone to oily skin and breakouts in this decade, so if this is a problem get into the habit of cleansing your face twice a day with a product that contains salicylic acid to unblock pores, reduce inflammation and keep spots at bay.
- A healthy, balanced diet with plenty of fresh fruit and veg will keep your body working well and give you the vital vitamins and minerals you need to promote healthy skin, hair and nails. For advice on diet, see pages 58–65.
- If your skin is greasy, don't use harsh products containing alcohol, as they will dry out the skin surface, and this will actually make you produce more oil to try to compensate for the dryness.

Beauty bag must-haves

- A non-greasy, oil-free moisturiser will ensure skin stays soft without exacerbating oiliness and causing spots. Oil-free means it won't block pores but it will still hydrate your skin where it's needed. Dermalogica Oil Control Lotion works really well.
- If you want some coverage, I'm a big fan of mineral make up, which is actually good for your skin. It's like skincare with colour. The molecules in the make-up are too large to be absorbed, so it won't clog pores even if you forget to wash it off after a late night. It also has the added benefit of a natural physical sunscreen of

around SPF 20 as it contains finely ground titanium dioxide and zinc oxide that give full-spectrum sun protection. My favourite brands are BPC and Mineral Earth, which you can order online. (For more great mineral make-up tips, see page 92.)

- Your lips are at their fullest in your 20s, so all you need is a slick of lip balm or moisturising gloss to protect your youthful pout.
- Let's face it, most people look better with a little bit of a tan, but please don't sunbathe or use sunbeds – it's the fastest way to get wrinkles and increases your risk of skin cancer. Just fake it or try a light dusting of bronzer across your cheekbones and temples, where the sun would naturally hit your face.
- Play up your natural youthful glow with a little pink blush applied with a large make-up brush to the apples (the round bit when you smile) of your cheeks. This is also great for hiding the effects of too many late nights.

BODY

You're at your physical peak right now and may feel you don't need to bother exercising. This is a big mistake because you'll find it harder to acquire the habit later on when exercise becomes more crucial to maintaining your body weight.

Steer clear of faddy crash diets or you'll be setting yourself up for a lifetime of yo-yo dieting, which isn't healthy. You might lose a ton of weight consuming nothing but cabbage soup, but you'll put it all back on again as soon as you start eating normally. Try to eat well 80% of the time and treat yourself the other 20%.

Body boosters
- Develop a water habit: be sure to drink plenty of water each day to keep your body hydrated and flush out any toxins.

- Try to eat five or six portions of fruit and veg a day to ensure you're getting plenty of health-boosting vitamins and minerals. If you get into the habit now, a balanced diet should become second nature as you get older.
- Watch the booze: all things in moderation should be every 20-something's motto. Party by all means, but go easy on the habits that can cause lifelong damage.
- Having said that, avoid smoking. You'll be glad you didn't succumb when you see your smoking friends developing crow's feet and little smoker's grooves along their top lips in their 30s, while you are still wrinkle-free.
- Get moving: take advantage of your fitness and high energy levels, and enjoy more adventurous forms of exercise such as snow-boarding, kickboxing and dancing.

GET AN ATTITUDE!

At this age you're probably at your most self-critical and lacking in confidence, but don't let your insecurities get the better of you. Enjoy your youth and put your boundless energy to good use, setting up healthy habits that will last a lifetime.

These are the 'try-out' years, so don't be afraid to test lots of different haircuts, make-up trends and clothes to find the styles that suit you. You'll have loads of fun along the way.

Your 30s

You may look and feel at your prime in this decade, but changes are afoot as your metabolism slows and the skin's natural collagen and elastin decline. The way you respond to these changes will affect the way you age in the decades to come.

SKIN

When women come to me for advice, I always ask them at what age they looked their absolute best, and virtually all of them say in their mid to late 30s. Certainly for me, by that age I'd sussed out what suited me, had a little more cash for good skincare products and generally felt a lot more confident.

The 30s is also the decade when you start to notice some crinkling and puffiness around your eyes, and that your cheeks look a little flatter. The skin's natural collagen and elastin that have kept your skin so supple begin to break down and faint expression lines start to form. If you've not been using sunscreen, the damage may start to become visible.

Thankfully, there's plenty you can still do to slow the ageing process and maintain a fresh-faced look.

Skin savers
- Continue to cleanse and moisturise twice daily to get rid of the dirt and pollution that clog pores and to keep skin hydrated. Don't forget to wear a sunscreen or SPF make-up every day. For more on good daily skincare, see page 31.
- Switch to a moisturiser with added anti-ageing ingredients such as retinol, antioxidants and hyaluronic acid to start fighting fine lines. See pages 110–32 for lots of tips on anti-ageing skincare.
- Take your skincare products down to your neck and décolletage; the skin in these areas is delicate and often exposed to sunshine, and therefore more prone to ageing.

- Counteract the dulling effect of slower skin renewal by using exfoliators that contain alpha hydroxy acids (AHAs). They can help keep skin youthful and radiant by getting rid of all those dead skin cells that dull your complexion and make lines appear deeper.

- This might be the decade to start paying a little more attention to the skin around your eyes to help keep crow's feet at bay. Eye gels and light serums are best as they won't cause puffiness. Apply them by gently tapping the product around the orbital bone. For more great tips on younger-looking eyes, see pages 134–45.

- If you want to improve the texture of your skin so it appears smoother, less crinkly and more luminous, it's worth talking to a dermatologist about procedures such as light chemical peels or microdermabrasion. These will freshen the surface of your skin and reduce fine lines. If you're looking for quicker, more dramatic results, it's worth considering a little Botox towards the end of this decade to help reduce the appearance of deeper wrinkles. See pages 133–78 for lots of advice on non-surgical anti-ageing treatments.

Beauty bag must-haves

- Now is the time to invest in skincare products with vitamin-A derivative retinol, which will boost radiance and smooth fine lines. Skin Doctors Retanew is a good one to try and can be found in Boots.

- Your skin may have lost a little of its natural glow and late nights may leave more traces on the face than they used to, so invest in a good tinted moisturiser as an alternative to foundation to warm up washed-out skin. I like Laura Mercier Tinted Moisturiser SPF 20.

- If dark circles are starting to plague you, it's time to get your hands on that celebrity favourite – a light-reflecting concealer. YSL's Touche Éclat is the gold standard, but there are many similar versions.

- Even if you're a super-busy mum and have no time for make-up, brush on some mascara before you leave the house. It will make you look wide awake and perk up your eyes. Maybelline Great Lash Mascara is the world's best-selling brand; it's great value and gives good results.

BODY

In your 30s your metabolism starts to slow down and you'll notice that it's becoming harder to shift those extra pounds. If you don't exercise, your metabolism will slow further and your muscle tone will start to decline and bones thin, increasing your risk of osteoporosis (also known as brittle bone disease). Many women who become mums in their 30s find they never shift the pregnancy weight, which only adds to the problem. If you haven't already done so in your 20s, this is the decade to get a healthy diet and exercise plan underway. It only gets harder the longer you leave it!

Body boosters
- Eat oily fish. The Omega 3 fats contained in oily fish such as salmon and mackerel can help boost skin condition and promote healthy hair and nails, so try to eat one or preferably two portions each week.
- Get off the sofa. If you've never been one for exercise, now is definitely the time to start. Absolutely nothing beats regular cardio workouts to keep you fit and toned and your body looking younger. Swimming, cycling or jogging three times a week will do the trick.
- But don't become a gym junkie. Some women in their 30s go too far and become addicted to exercise in a bid to stay young.

Overdoing it actually has the opposite effect, leaving you skinny and stealing much-needed volume from your face and cheeks. Working out for between 30 and 45 minutes three times a week is plenty.

- Lose that baby weight. The key for new mothers is to stick to a healthy, gradual weight-loss plan that aims to shift the weight slowly, but keep it off for good.

See pages 218–19 for some exercises that will help you to trim up your waistline and flatten your tummy again.

GET AN ATTITUDE!

For a lot of women, the 30s are the 'arriving' years. Many of us settle down to married bliss, have a baby or get that dream job, and any one of these achievements can create an inner glow that money just can't buy. You're much more confident in who you are and where you're going in life, and this can be the decade when you have the drive to get what you want without worrying about what others think.

You'll also have developed your personal style and worked out what suits you, so make the most of it.

Your 40s

Ah, the fabulous 40s! You've grown into your looks, you have bags more confidence, and you also have the means to do something about your appearance if you don't like it.

SKIN

In my experience a woman's skin changes more in this decade than any other. Although it may still look healthy and vibrant, the effects of long-term sun exposure, repetitive facial expressions and the normal ageing process will become apparent as the decade advances. The rate at which your skin is renewing itself has slowed down so those once-fine lines around your eyes and mouth start to deepen and forehead lines may begin to appear.

Around this time women also experience hormonal changes as oestrogen and progesterone levels decline in the run-up to the menopause. This in turn triggers a drop in collagen and elastin production so skin loses some of its spring, and there is less production of sebum (skin oil) leading to drier, thinner skin.

It can sometimes seem as if skin loses its youthfulness, plumpness and tone overnight – but don't panic. There's still plenty of opportunity to maintain a radiant complexion and delay those lines and wrinkles with the right skincare regime.

Skin savers

- Continue to use a high SPF moisturiser daily and, if you're not already doing so, start using one that contains anti-ageing ingredients such as retinol, AHAs and antioxidants. (I've de-jargoned all of these 'miracle' anti-ageing ingredients on pages 110–30.) In my view an anti-ageing cream that contains vitamin-A derivative retinol is a must for women in their 40s. Retinol boosts skin turnover and collagen production and gives you back some of that radiance you've lost. These days, most good anti-ageing creams contain it.
- If your skin is dull, try an at-home microdermabrasion product to reveal a more youthful glow. This is an exfoliator that uses tiny beads to mechanically remove dead skin cells, and it will help to even out skin tone and improve texture. Try No7 Total Renewal

Micro-Dermabrasion from Boots. Glycolic peels at a salon work in a similar way but will have a more dramatically rejuvenating effect. See page 167 for all you need to know about peels.

- Try to schedule a facial treatment once a month, but choose one that's results driven rather than just a nice relaxing deep cleanse. Go for a facial that uses massage (to boost circulation and deliver nutrients to the skin), microdermabrasion (to get rid of dead skin cells that dull your complexion) and proven anti-ageing ingredients such as glycolic acid (to boost cell renewal for a more even, luminous complexion). See Chapter 6 for descriptions of lots of great DIY anti-ageing treatments.

- If non-surgical 'helpers' are within your budget, now is probably the time to start. Better to have a little now than a lot later. A little Botox on your forehead can knock off five years instantly by taking away those angry frown furrows and tired-looking lines. Hyaluronic acid fillers can also plump out wrinkles around your mouth. See pages 137 and 158.

Beauty bag must-haves

- Get an antioxidant-rich moisturiser with an SPF of at least 15 for use during the day.

- Every morning apply a light hydrating eye cream (the most important ingredient is an SPF). Dermalogica makes a good one called Total Eyecare, which also contains light-reflecting pigments to minimise dark circles.

- Every evening, apply a serum. These have a lighter consistency than regular creams and are absorbed more easily into the skin. Make sure it contains retinol to boost skin cell turnover. Try MD Formulations VitAPlus Anti-Aging Serum or Lancôme Visionnaire Advanced Skin Corrector.

- Dark circles get more prominent with age so it's important to invest in a concealer specifically for use under the eyes. Choose a wand-style one that has a lighter consistency so it won't sit in fine lines, making them more visible.

- If your eyelashes have become sparse, opt for falsies for a night out or start using a volumising mascara.

BODY

Even women who don't normally put on a pound in weight may now expand in size. After 40 virtually all women find that they gain fat more easily – below the bra, through the triceps area (those cursed bingo wings), on the back, and on the tummy. You're not doing anything wrong; it's just that your body composition is changing, and you need to adjust your diet and exercise regime accordingly. You'll be more prone to injury than you were in your 30s so don't overdo the exercise. Strength training such as squats, lunges, press-ups and crunches will help to speed up your waning metabolism and keep you toned.

For each decade after the age of 40, your body needs 5% fewer calories – but don't despair. You can easily drop these 100 calories a day by cutting out one of your daily snacks.

Body boosters

- Eat oestrogen-mimicking foods. Pulses, bean sprouts, flaxseeds (linseeds) and green, leafy vegetables will all help to counter the effects of the drop in oestrogen your body is experiencing.
- Oily fish such as salmon can help combat middle-aged spread as they contain the protein leptin, which acts like a hormone, reducing fat storage around your middle and controlling your appetite so you don't overeat.
- To avoid the post-40 spread you need to be exercising at least three times a week, for 45 minutes a time, to a level where you're a little out of breath and starting to sweat.

- <u>Start pumping iron!</u> Lifting light arm and leg weights will keep your limbs toned and help increase muscle mass, keeping your metabolic rate as high as possible, so you stay slim.

GET AN ATTITUDE!

I think this could be described as the 'sexy decade'! Women in their early 40s seem to exude more sex appeal than in any other decade. Maybe it's that final flush of fertility before the menopause or just their wonderful self-confidence. Be sure to harness it!

You're probably as busy as ever, juggling work with looking after kids, but no matter how hectic things are, be a little selfish and reserve some time for yourself and your partner.

Your 50s

Nobody ever said life was fair. Just as your waist reaches its thickest point, your face starts to get thinner and look older. It's all down to those pesky hormones again as oestrogen levels continue to plummet in your sixth decade, but fortunately there's plenty you can do to counteract the changes taking place. Get it right and this could become your best beauty decade so far!

SKIN

Most women are by now in the thick of the menopause, which we know damages skin elasticity, firmness and moisture levels. Your skin will probably feel drier and saggier as a result and you may begin to see much more prominent wrinkles around your mouth, forehead and eyes, while the face and neck become saggy and jowly. Hands can also become blotchy and the skin on the neck and décolletage becomes thinner, with more age spots and wrinkles.

But take heart! Your 50s can be the time to fight back and repair sagging skin. It's crucial that you are completely consistent with your skincare in order to achieve lasting benefits.

Skin savers
- Continue using a high SPF suncream daily. Take extra care in the sun and you can still reap some rewards in terms of slowing down sun damage and perhaps even repairing some of it.
- Using skincare products containing glycolic acid will help trigger new cell growth and collagen formation over time, as well as aiding exfoliation.
- Try a chemical peel – these can shave off years in less than an hour by removing the damaged top layers of your skin.
- If you have very badly sun-damaged skin, a dermatologist may prescribe Retin-A, a powerful vitamin-A cream. It'll help reduce fine lines and wrinkles, improve skin texture and tone and fade sun spots. You can't use it all the time, though, as your skin will become flaky and red (a bit like having facial dandruff). I'd recommend using it every other night for a week, once every few months.
- If skincare isn't cutting it, this might be the time to consider fillers to plump up certain areas of the face, restoring a youthful fullness.

Beauty bag must-haves
- Fake a plump, youthful pout by using a nude lip pencil around the outer lip line (it'll help prevent lipstick bleed, too). Bobbi Brown has a great range of neutral colours to suit every skin tone.
- Choose creamy or moisturising lipsticks and avoid matte textures, which can make lips look drier and older. Estée Lauder Signature Hydra Lustre Lipstick keeps lips super-smooth.

- Pearly shades of eyeshadow will sit unflatteringly in the lines around your eyes and highlight crêpey skin. Go for a cream or satin finish.
- Since mature skin tends to be drier, choose a light, moisturising foundation that keeps skin hydrated and won't sit in wrinkles.
- Even if you've worn it all your life, red lipstick can be too harsh for older skins and pile on the years, so stick to paler pinks and neutral shades for a softer look. For lots of clever ideas on how to de-age your make-up bag, see pages 88–96.

BODY

No matter how slim they are, women tend to gain a little pot belly at this age, as hormone levels ensure they store more fat than they burn off. But sticking to a healthy diet and continuing to exercise will pay dividends.

Body boosters

- Levels of friendly bacteria in the gut drop after the age of 50 leaving you at increased risk of a sluggish digestion and bloating. A poor digestion means you're not absorbing the nutrients from food effectively, and these are needed for a healthy body and skin function. The result – you look and feel older! Drinking a probiotic drink or eating some live yoghurt every day will help combat this.
- Nibbling nuts can help shift tummy fat, as they're high in protein and essential fatty acids, along with vitamin E, which can help you feel fuller for longer, balance your hormones and ward off sugar cravings. They contain lots of calories, though, so nibble in moderation!

- Research shows that middle-aged women who eat wholegrain bread and brown rice along with wholegrain pasta and cereals tend to have smaller waistlines than those who get exactly the same number of calories from white carbs. It's well worth swapping over.

- Improve your posture. Try this stretch to banish stooping. Clasp your hands behind your back at bottom level and squeeze your shoulder blades together. Straighten your arms and gently try to stretch your fingertips towards the floor until you notice a light tug between your ears and shoulders. Finally lift your hands as high above your head as you can, feeling the stretch in your chest.

- Easy does it! It's important to be active in your 50s but if you haven't exercised for a long time, do start slowly. In the US they've coined the phrase 'boomeritis' to describe the common injuries they see as a result of middle-aged people suddenly taking to exercise a little too energetically. Aim for four 30-minutes bouts of moderate activity – such as brisk walking, swimming or dance classes – every week.

GET AN ATTITUDE!

You may be feeling emotional, thanks to the menopause – yes, there'll be tears a teenager would be proud of! But you'll also have gained maturity and wisdom and will have worked out your priorities. You'll be a lot more relaxed and now the kids are big and ugly enough to look after themselves, you'll have a lot more time to focus on yourself and your relationship with your partner. Make the most of this new-found freedom and try new hobbies, take more holidays and enjoy yourself. This decade can be filled with fun and laughter.

Your 60s and beyond

Take good care of yourself now and you'll stay looking and feeling as fabulous as 60-something role models Susan Sarandon, who puts her amazing looks down to quitting smoking and doing Pilates every day, and Helen Mirren, who swears by her beauty sleep and a sensible diet.

SKIN

After two decades of changes, your hormones will have finally settled down, which means your skin should become more stable. Wrinkles, red veins and dark spots are common, but they will be less pronounced provided you've got into the habit of protecting your skin from the sun in previous decades.

Your skin is likely to be thinner and drier now than it used to be, which can make it more vulnerable to environmental damage and more prone to irritation. You may find you become sensitive to products you've used all your life. The best approach to daily skincare is therefore to use gentle, hydrating products twice a day that protect and add much-needed moisture.

Skin savers
- Once you are post-menopausal, you can use products that contain natural progesterone and oestrogen to improve your skin's firmness and elasticity. Try creams such as Jan Marini Age Intervention Face Cream or B. Kamins Therapeutic Diamond Radiance Deep Wrinkle Concentrate.
- Keep up good skincare habits. Use a gentle hydrating cleanser, along with a good anti-ageing moisturiser that contains an SPF. Gently exfoliate twice a week to increase the cell renewal

rate and maintain a fresher, healthier glow. Don't stop at your neck; exfoliate your whole body, paying a little more attention to feet, elbows and the tops of your arms. For a gentler exfoliation, try using a flannel instead of an exfoliation product. And keep skin silky-soft by using a body lotion every day after your bath or shower.

- Choose a new hair colour (wisely). Opt for softer tones, because anything too vibrant or too dark can leave your skin looking washed out.

- Tackle age spots. Most of the creams you can buy at the local pharmacy aren't strong enough to fade pigmentation, but a dermatologist or a cosmetic doctor will be able to prescribe a cream that has enough power to erase them.

- If good skincare isn't enough, ask your dermatologist or a cosmetic doctor about chemical peels and laser procedures, which will remove multiple layers of dead skin cells and might just create the dramatic difference you're searching for. See pages 166–8 and 191–2 for advice on these treatments.

Beauty bag must-haves

- Regular spritzing can help mature skins stay hydrated. Rosewater in particular is great for refreshing skin; try Barefoot Botanicals Rosa Fina Facial Spritz.

- It's not just your face that gives away your age. Prune-like hands will reveal your birthday quicker than anything else, so invest in a good anti-ageing hand cream that helps tackle sun spots. If your hands are letting the side down, think about a clinic treatment to restore some youthful plumpness and get rid of age spots. For more on this, see pages 209–15.

- A skin serum used regularly can help firm and nourish skin. Try Caudalie Vinexpert Firming Serum.

- If your eyebrows have become thinner, redefine them with a good-quality brow-defining pencil in a shade that's not too dark. If greys are the problem, get them professionally dyed and shaped at a salon.

BODY

Many people find their appetite changes after 60 and you may benefit from eating little and often instead of three big meals a day. But it's more important than ever to eat a healthy diet as the slimmer you remain, the more active you'll stay in these decades.

Your natural posture and balance can start to decline, leading to stooping, so it's vital to stick to a gentle exercise regime to keep your body strong and supple and to burn off excess calories. But don't overdo it – it's worth talking to a fitness coach about adapting your workout routine as you enter your 60s, as you may need to ease off on any exercises that might jar and stress your joints.

Body boosters
- Wear and tear on your digestive system can mean bloating and constipation become more of a problem for 60-somethings. Combat this by eating more fibre-rich fruit and veg and whole-grain bread.
- Take up yoga or tai chi; both are gentle workouts that improve posture and balance.
- Swimming or riding a stationary bicycle are both great low-impact activities that will keep you fit without jarring joints.
- If you don't stretch daily in your 60s, by the time you are in your 70s and 80s your joints will have lost their flexibility. The old

adage 'use it or lose it' holds true here, so start each day with a few simple warm-up stretches, such as the following:

- To stretch your neck, sit or stand with your arms loose by your sides, then gently tilt your head, first to one side, then the other, holding for five seconds each side.
- To warm up the back of your neck, tilt your head forwards and hold for five seconds.
- To target your shoulders and upper arms, bring one arm right across your chest and place your hand on the opposite shoulder, hold for ten to 15 seconds then repeat on the other side.
- To warm up shoulders, middle back, arms and hands, clasp your hands together in front of you, then turn your palms so they're facing away from you and stretch your arms out in front of you at shoulder height. Hold for ten to 20 seconds, then repeat.
- To stretch the waist, backs of arms and tops of shoulders, lift your arms above your head (you can be sitting or standing). Hold your left elbow with your right hand, then gently pull your left elbow over your head as you slowly lean to the right. Hold for ten to 15 seconds then repeat on the other side.
- To warm up your middle back, stand with your feet hip-width apart, knees slightly bent. With hands on hips, gently twist your torso at the waist until you feel a mild stretch. Hold for ten to 15 seconds then repeat on the other side.
- To get your ankles working, sit in a chair and lift one foot off the floor, rotate your ankle eight to ten times clockwise, then eight to ten times anti-clockwise. Repeat with the other foot.
- To stretch the fronts of your thighs, place your left hand on a wall in front of you for support, then grab your left foot with your right hand and pull it gently towards your bottom. Hold for ten to 20 seconds, then repeat on the other side.

- To warm up the backs of your legs and your lower back, sit on the floor with your legs in front of you in a V shape. Bend your left leg in at the knee, then slowly lean forward from your hips towards your right foot until you feel a mild stretch. Don't let your head drop down. Hold for ten to 20 seconds, then repeat on the other side.

GET AN ATTITUDE!

You can still be fabulous in your 60s and beyond. It's up to you. You can opt to be a 'Glamma' (a glamorous granny) or you can settle for a twin-set and a pair of comfy shoes. I know what I'd prefer. You have more freedom, money and time to focus on your needs at this age, and it's great to be able to pick and choose when to see the kids and grandchildren.

Now's the time to consider cosmetic surgery if you really want to turn back the clock. I knew a lady who had a face-lift in her 70s because she finally had the cash, and it gave her a whole new lease of life. On the other hand, my mum has never had any surgical help and she's still gorgeous because her naughty personality shines through. The point is, we have choices and there's plenty of advice later in the book to help you choose wisely.

two
Love the Skin You're In

Before you even think about anti-ageing treatments, the first thing to do is get your skin into tip-top condition, and that's what this chapter is all about. We're talking about good skincare habits for a healthy complexion, combatting problems such as blemishes and rosacea, getting rid of all that nasty unwanted body hair and, the most important one of all, protecting your skin from its greatest enemy – the sun!

The fact is, we chuck a lot of stuff at our skin every day and just expect it to bounce right back and look amazing. The skin on our face is under attack from the weather, drying central heating, grimy city air – not to mention bombarded by toxins from alcohol, cigarettes and processed foods. Phew! So it really pays to treat it to some TLC.

With that in mind, the most important thing you can do for your skin is care for it on a daily basis. In my opinion it's much better for your skin to find the right products to use at home, and get into a routine of using them every day, than to spend a fortune on a facial once a month.

I'm always surprised by the number of women coming to my clinic for a consultation who, when I ask them to describe their beauty regime, tell me it doesn't really exist. A half-hearted cleanse followed by a quick slick of any old moisturiser is about as good as it gets. Exfoliation is a once-in-a-blue-moon treat!

But cleansing is one area you shouldn't skimp on. Take your time, enjoy a few minutes to reflect on the day ahead or the day you've just had, and enjoy the feeling of really clean skin. Here's my step-by-step guide.

A clean sweep

To avoid being 'too tired' to cleanse properly at night so you end up falling into bed with all your make-up on, do your beauty routine as soon as you get home in the evening if you're not going out anywhere. It's a good way to wind down from work or a busy day, and you'll have more time for add-ons such as face masks or exfoliation.

STEP 1

Apply your cleanser to your face and neck, massaging it upwards and paying special attention to the chin and the area around your nose. Taking a couple of minutes for a little massage like this twice a day while you're cleansing will boost blood flow, delivering nutrients to your skin.

Choose a simple cleanser that won't irritate your skin. My favourite is Cetaphil Gentle Skin Cleanser, which you'll find in Boots. Beauty

> **TIP!** Occasionally washing your face with egg yolk will help to stimulate your skin a little, boosting cell turnover. The magic ingredient is vitamin A. After removing make-up with your regular cleanser, apply the egg yolk all over your face with a cotton pad, avoiding the eye area. Leave on for about five minutes, then rinse off with warm water. Easy!

experts love this little product because it suits all skin types and it's particularly good if you have acne or sensitive skin as it won't strip the skin of its natural oils or disrupt its pH balance. I prefer wash-off cleansers because creamy lotions that you wipe off with cotton pads often leave a film on the skin.

Don't forget to exfoliate!

If you're using a flannel every day to take off your cleanser, that will help to slough away dead skin cells, but amazingly they come back after only 11 hours! You can use a moisturiser or serum that contains alpha hydroxy acids (AHAs), which will exfoliate your skin every day, but this can be too much for some people.

My advice would be to use an exfoliation product twice a week. Some granular exfoliators can be very harsh and scratch the skin, so make sure you choose a product that contains jojoba spheres, diamond dust, salt or oats, which are all gentle on the skin. I like Jurlique Daily Exfoliating Cream, which contains oats, almonds and honey.

I use an exfoliator I developed myself (Microdermabrasion With Crushed Diamonds), which also has the AHA glycolic acid in it. I put it on my face before I jump in the shower, making sure it's the last thing I wash off before I get out, so the glycolic acid has had a little time to work its magic and dissolve the 'glue' that holds the dead cells together.

Exfoliation is very important because by getting rid of dead cells on the surface of your skin, it not only makes lines appear less obvious, but it also allows the anti-ageing ingredients in your face cream to penetrate and work more effectively.

TIP! For a gentle home-made exfoliator, mix together some runny honey and oats. Apply the mixture to your face and massage in gently, using small circular movements. Leave on for a minute or two, then rinse off with a flannel and warm water, and pat dry with a clean towel. This also makes a good exfoliator for dry, flaky lips.

STEP 2

Always take your cleanser off with a flannel that's been soaked in warm water, as this will help to remove dead skin cells. Rinsing with water alone will leave all those dead cells on the surface of your skin, making your complexion look dull and wrinkles appear deeper. For extra exfoliation, gently rub your skin dry with a clean, dry flannel. Remember to wash flannels every couple of days to get rid of any bacteria.

We're always being told to cleanse, tone and moisturise, but toners are a waste of money. If you cleanse your face properly, you don't need them. Many toners also contain alcohol, which strips skin of its natural oils, leaving it dry, so your skin produces more oil to compensate. If you like the fresh feeling of a toner, look for one that doesn't contain alcohol or, better still, use a spritz of rosewater when you feel your skin needs freshening up. Rosewater has anti-inflammatory properties so is good for all skin types and is particularly beneficial for drier, more mature complexions. The fragrance is uplifting, too!

STEP 3

Apply your moisturiser, but only where it's needed, say on your cheeks, around your eyes and over your top lip. Pat it on to your face so your skin absorbs as much as possible rather than trying to rub it in, as rubbing will probably result in wiping most of it off.

If you're lucky enough to have fantastic skin, you may be able to get away with a good natural face cream. Brands to check out are Dr Hauschka (its Rose Day Cream Light is a firm celebrity favourite), Jurlique and Caudalie. Just make sure you go for a light formula. However, if you want a cream that does more than simply hydrate, turn to page 110 for my advice on the best anti-ageing ingredients to look for in a moisturiser.

Closing open pores

Many of the women I see at my clinic are bothered by open pores. These are pores clogged with dead skin cells, oil, make-up and general dirt and they can leave your skin looking uneven and grubby. They show up as blackheads when the pore is blocked and the sebum at the surface oxidises so it looks black. When pores become full they stretch so they look large and wide open. It's a bit like stuffing too much into a hand-bag and not being able to close the zip!

The quickest DIY fix is a steam facial. Run hot water into a bowl, cover your head with a towel to trap the steam and place your face above

> **TIP!** There are a few clever products that minimise the appearance of enlarged pores, such as my own Harley Street Skin Microdermabrasion or the Dr Brandt Pores No More range. You could also try BPC loose oat powder in Buff. This is an excellent product that you dot on with a brush before applying foundation to minimise the appearance of pores. I use it myself.

What you DO and DON'T want in your beauty products

It pays to limit chemical overload in the products you're regularly putting on your skin, particularly if it's sensitive and prone to allergies and breakouts. Therefore, try to limit the use of products containing the following, where possible:

- Sodium lauryl/laureth sulfate – this is very drying but it's used in lots of foaming face cleansers and is a common cause of irritation. If you notice a rash or redness after using a cleanser containing it, stop using it.
- Mineral oil – this is an inexpensive by-product of petroleum and is used in lots of lotions, creams and cosmetics. It forms a barrier on the skin, clogging pores and preventing natural oils in the skin from coming out, so it helps spots to form. Avoid it!
- Chemical fragrances – these are often a cause of allergies and skin irritations such as hives, rashes and dermatitis. Look for natural fragrances such as essential oils or choose fragrance-free products.
- Parabens – these are commonly used in moisturising creams as a preservative and can cause skin rashes and irritation. Look for products that include a natural preservative instead.
- Alcohols (including ethanol, ethyl alcohol, and isopropyl) – these are very drying and irritating, disturbing the skin's natural pH and making it more vulnerable to bacteria, fungi and viruses. Don't go there!

What you do want

- Your day cream should include an SPF, but if your favourite brand doesn't have one, make sure you apply sunscreen on top or use a foundation or tinted moisturiser with SPF 15. Mineral make-up contains a natural sunscreen (see page 91).
- For the lowdown on the best anti-ageing ingredients to look for in a moisturiser, see page 111.

the water. After a few minutes of steaming, the pores will begin to open enough to loosen the dead skin, oil and dirt that has been blocking them. Now you can use a gentle exfoliating facial scrub to get rid of the debris. Finish by rinsing your face with cold water. Repeat this steam facial once a week or as often as needed.

Some people like to squeeze their blackheads to unclog the pores, but they tend to keep filling up with sebum and dead skin cells unless you regularly use a gentle AHA serum. Apply it once a week if your skin is sensitive or every day if you have an oily or very sun-damaged complexion. Adding a detoxifying face mask to your beauty routine once a week can help.

The most important thing to keep pore problems at bay is to cleanse your face properly twice a day and exfoliate twice a week.

Banish those blemishes for good!

OK, let's get something straight: acne has nothing to do with being dirty. It's caused by hormones (the male ones) that stimulate oil production. Although we associate it with puberty, it can affect you at any time in your life if hormones are out of balance. I got a spot on the end of my nose the day before my wedding! Fortunately, I was marrying a cosmetic surgeon, so I asked him to give me a 'spot' injection of cortisone and it disappeared within 24 hours.

Your skin-type tips

If you have...

- Sensitive skin – patch test products before you buy them and choose skincare that isn't overloaded with chemicals. Try natural, organic brands and go for the simplest formulas you can find. Chemical suncreens often cause sensitivity, so opt for barrier sunblocks that use minerals such as zinc oxide.
- Dry skin – in winter, central heating can leave skin even more parched than normal, so pop a bowl of water on the radiator or on a surface nearby to let some moisture evaporate into the air. Don't over-exfoliate with harsh scrubs. Choose a gentle product and use it once a week only. 'Moisturise' your skin from the inside with an Omega 3, 6 and 9 supplement (see page 64).
- Oily skin – never be tempted to use a harsh toner; in the long run it'll make your skin produce even more oil. Only use moisturiser where it's needed and avoid the oily T-zone. Go for creams and suncare products that are non-comedogenic – that means they won't block pores.
- Combination skin – avoid moisturising the T-zone, which will probably be oily, and give a little extra hydration to your cheeks, which will probably be dry. Use different face masks for each of these areas: a deep cleansing and detoxifying one for the T-zone and a moisturising one for your cheeks.

There are different forms of acne, but all of them cause a great deal of distress for sufferers. It can totally wreck your confidence and self-esteem. In the clinic we see between six and eight cases every day, and sometimes those clients have put up with it for ten years or more.

Luckily for the women who come to my clinic, acne is a pet subject of mine. I started focusing on it when my son Adam became covered in pimples when he was about 14 so it looked as though he had a red, bumpy rash. I used mild glycolic peels on him – in those days there was little available other than antibiotics in the UK – and made him stick to a skincare routine. The spots upset him so much that he followed my advice religiously until the acne started to clear – but sure enough within a week it would erupt again. That's the problem with acne. You have to hang in there when treating it.

For me, the acne drug Roaccutane is off the agenda – I don't like it. It's been linked to thinning of the skin, bleeding, even depression. There are lots of other ways you can clear acne, with perseverance, support and the right products and (perhaps) medicines.

There are varying degrees of acne – from whiteheads and blackheads to nodules and cysts – so here's what to look out for and how to treat it.

- Whiteheads (medically known as closed comedones) are formed when pores are blocked, so the oil produced by the skin (sebum) is trapped inside along with dead skin cells. Bacteria then grow and, as the pore becomes more blocked and over-filled, you see a small white raised lump on the surface of the skin.
- Blackheads (medically known as open comedones), which we've already discussed in relation to open pores, are at the very mild end of the scale but they can often take a long time to clear.
- Papules are inflamed, red, sore bumps with no head. I know it's tempting, but DON'T squeeze a papule, as it can leave a nasty scar.

- Pustules are inflamed red spots with a white or yellow centre. These 'zits' can be popped, but only when they are ready to burst! Pop them with a sterile needle, then wrap a clean tissue around each of your index fingers and squeeze gently. It's best to do this after a warm shower or facial steaming as they'll be softer. If clear liquid or blood starts to appear, it is time to stop squeezing!

- Nodules are large, hard, painful bumps under the skin, which often last for months. Never squeeze them as this can cause permanent scarring. The best thing you can do is to have them injected with cortisone (as I had before my wedding). Cortisone is produced naturally in the body, so you won't have a reaction. It works by killing bacteria and reducing inflammation. It's something we do on a regular basis at our clinic. Many celebrities pop in to have a spot injected so it retreats speedily before a red-carpet event. Now you know about it, you can ask for it, too. Alternatively, dab them with a little HSS Glyco Serum – another celeb favourite.

- Cysts look similar to nodules, except they are full of pus – yuck! They are usually very painful and can leave scarring. Squeezing cysts can cause a deep irritation and very painful inflammation, which will last much longer than if you had left it alone. Once again, the cortisone 'spot' injection can help and I promise your cyst will be gone in a maximum of 48 hours.

MY ACNE CLEAR-UP PLAN

Follow this plan to clear acne from your face, chest and/or back – wherever your skin is affected.

1. Use a gentle product to clean your skin, such as my favourite, Cetaphil Gentle Skin Cleanser. Resist the urge to scrub as this will

leave skin dry and flaky and your body will try to counteract the dryness by producing more oil.

2. Wash off your cleanser with a flannel to stop dead skin cells becoming trapped in pores. Use a clean flannel every day and pat your face dry with a paper towel.

3. Apply an AHA serum. I like glycolic acid because it's very effective at getting rid of dead skin cells and is gentle, too. NeoStrata, Jan Marini or HSS are all good brands to try.

4. Apply an oil-free moisturiser – again Cetaphil is inexpensive and excellent. You need a moisturiser even though you have oily skin, as you'll still have dry patches. Just apply it where it's needed.

5. Use sunscreen daily to protect your skin and prevent pigmentation marks after spots clear up.

6. At night dab benzoyl peroxide cream on spots with a cotton bud. Let it dry before it comes into contact with pyjamas, bed sheets and towels or the peroxide will bleach them. Benzoyl peroxide is available over the counter, but your doctor can prescribe a higher-strength version.

7. Take a supplement of Omega 3, 6 and 9 oils to nourish your skin from the inside (see page 64).

8. Find ways to reduce stress, as it stimulates the production of androgens – the hormones that stimulate oil. For tips on this, see pages 74–9.

9. If you keep touching your face, it'll just spread the bacteria. Resist the urge.

10. Don't be tempted to go on sunbeds or sunbathe to reduce acne – it'll only leave you with mauve or brown scarring.

For more severe, persistent acne, try the following:

• Have a course of light glycolic or salicylic acid peels at a clinic. These will get rid of dead skin cells for smoother, more even skin tone, and help diminish scarring. If you have bad scars, though, you might need to consider a laser resurfacing treatment, which does have an ouch factor (see pages 191–2).

- If your acne is severe or simply won't budge, see a dermatologist or cosmetic doctor about medication. Your doctor may suggest taking the contraceptive pill Dianette, but this can cause hyper-pigmention by stimulating melanin production, leaving you with unslightly brown marks across your forehead and top lip – lovely! There are alternatives that can reduce the impact of acne-causing hormones on your skin. The topical antibiotic Zineryt is excellent when used alongside a skincare routine that includes AHAs and benzoyl peroxide.

- Ask your doctor about a prescription for Retin-A. This vitamin A treatment is effective at boosting skin renewal and reducing oil production, but it must be used with care as it can make skin red and flaky if overused. You must also wear sunscreen to protect the newer skin from sun damage.

Coping with rosacea

This skin condition appears as a red rash on the cheeks, nose, forehead, eyelids and chin. It's more common in fair-skinned people, which is why it's nicknamed 'the curse of the Celts'. The redness is often accompanied by bumps or pimples (so it can be mistaken for acne) and sometimes skin can become dry, itchy and flaky, too.

Inflammation causes blood vessels to dilate so they become more visible, causing the red 'flushing' that characterises the condition – almost as if your skin is see-through.

Doctors still don't fully understand what causes rosacea, but 'flushing' appears to flare up with certain environmental factors, such as sun, exercise, spicy food, alcohol and some medications. I certainly believe that stress makes the condition worse.

It usually makes an appearance in the late 20s, although some women get it for the first time around the menopause.

WHAT YOU CAN DO

- It's useful to keep a diary to try and work out which triggers make your rosacea worse so you can do your best to avoid them.
- Look for a mild skincare range – again Cetaphil is good.
- Certain medications may help – there is a low-dose antibiotic called Efrasa, with which we've had great success at our clinic. You need to take it for around six months. And you could also ask whoever is treating you about allergy testing.
- Clinic treatments, including laser procedures or intense pulsed light (see pages 243–5), can work very well in reducing redness and visible blood vessels once the condition is under control.
- Only use mineral make-up, as it won't irritate the skin. It gives good coverage, too.

I've found we get the best results by using a combination of treatments, usually involving antibiotics and skincare products containing vitamin C, glycolic acid and antioxidants. It's also important to use sun protection. I like Avene High Protection Mineral Cream SPF 50, which is designed for intolerant skin.

Although rosacea responds to treatment, it may take weeks or months before you notice an improvement, so be patient. Papules and pustules tend to disappear quite quickly, but the redness and flushing will take longer.

Stay sun-safe

OK, let's be honest – we all love the feeling of being in the sun and most of us feel better when we have a bit of colour. But unfortunately, sun damage is *the* number-one cause of premature wrinkles. It's just not fair, is it? The single most important thing you can do to look after your skin and prevent premature ageing is to protect it from the sun. In fact, if you do nothing else for your skin except use a sunscreen for a year, it will improve.

The earlier you start using sun protection, the better. There's no doubt that if you start wearing a good sunscreen at 16, you'll be very grateful when you reach your 30s and 40s. My daughter Sophie is 17 and she's been using a daily sunscreen since she was about ten. I've always drummed the message home (she'll thank me for it later), but she also went to a very far-seeing school that wouldn't let the kids out to play in summer if they didn't have a sun hat and sun cream with them.

Every day, come rain or shine, it's vital to use a moisturiser or sun cream with SPF 15, although in high summer when you're outside for long periods, go for SPF 30. This is your very first step to slowing skin ageing.

When you're choosing a product, always go for a broad-spectrum sunscreen that protects against both UVA (long 'ageing' rays that penetrate the skin causing deep damage and ultimately wrinkles) and UVB (the shorter rays that give you sunburn). Of course, it's not just wrinkled skin we risk by being in the sun unprotected; there's the danger of skin cancer, too. And while we're on the subject of damaging UV light, never, ever use a sunbed, which also increases your risk of skin cancer and premature lines and is just as damaging as the sun.

There are lots of good sun-protection products on the market. I'm a fan of Australian brands because they've really had experience of protecting pale skin from sun damage. One of my favourites is Sunsense.

Always apply your sunscreen at least 15 minutes before leaving the house to allow it be absorbed properly. And if you're out for any length of time in strong sunlight, don't forget your sunglasses and a wide-brimmed hat.

TIP! If you've been following my advice, you won't risk getting sunburnt in the first place. However, if it happens, my tip is to add three capfuls of malt vinegar to a large bottle of still mineral water and keep it cool in the fridge. Dab it on to soothe sore or sunburnt skin.

Moles

If you have a lot of moles on your face or body, it's a good idea to get them checked yearly so any changes can be picked up. Moles or dark patches that are slightly raised or flat will usually remain harmless for your whole life. However, moles or patches of normal skin that change in size, shape or colour should be shown to your GP or dermatologist so they can rule out skin cancer. Other signs that can indicate skin cancer include a mole or spot that won't heal, hurts, itches or scabs. There are specialist clinics where you can have mole checks (such as the Mole Clinic in London – see page 281).

FAKE, DON'T BAKE!

If you just can't bear to be pale and interesting, the only safe way to get that golden glow is from a bottle. I always think the worst thing about fake tans is the smell, but these days that doesn't seem to be as much of a problem. The other issue is how to achieve a flawless streak-free finish when it's a DIY job. Here's my guide to getting the most natural look possible.

Prepare properly

For the best results, skin needs to be clean and smooth, so exfoliate your face and body in the shower first to smooth any dry, flaky areas of skin where the tan can collect giving a patchy finish. That means paying special attention to knees, elbows and the backs of your arms.

You also need to remove any hair from your top lip and chin (see pages 50–6), as this can trap excess tan – and an orange moustache isn't part of the plan! Pull your hair back from your face with a band to ensure you're blending the tan properly without leaving lines.

Shaving your legs after applying fake tan will make it streak and fade more quickly. It's a good idea to get your legs waxed so it'll be a few weeks before you next need to get rid of the hair.

Hydrate your skin

Your tan will go on more smoothly and easily if you moisturise beforehand, so apply your regular face cream and a liberal helping of body cream. Some sunless tanners don't have a great smell, so using a fragranced body cream is a good idea. Allow about 20 minutes for the cream to be absorbed, or your tan will just slide off and you'll risk a streaky finish.

Smooth it on

Don't squeeze the tan directly on to your body or face. Put some in your palms or on fingertips first and warm it before applying. Take care not to put too much tan around your eyebrows or hairline; use a damp cotton wool pad to remove any excess. Make sure you blend the tan under your jawline, down your neck and across your collarbone.

Use long sweeping movements to apply the tan to your body, taking care to blend evenly between fingers and toes and around the ankles. Again, you can remove any excess with damp cotton wool. Make sure you wash your hands thoroughly afterwards to avoid orange palms.

Let it develop

After you've applied your tan, throw on something loose like a beach kaftan (preferably not white!) to allow it to develop properly and ensure it's as patch-free as possible. Wait a couple of hours to see how you like the colour before another application. It's better to build the colour gradually.

> **TIP!** Remember that wearing fake tan won't protect your skin from the sun. Even if the one you buy contains sun protection factors, these will only be effective for a short time after you apply it. You still need to wear a good sunscreen with a high SPF.

Choosing fake tans

Here are three of my top sunless tanners…

- My favourite has to be Clarins Delicious Self Tanning Cream, which has a mousse-like texture and contains a touch of iridescent gold, giving you a lovely golden glow as well as a beautiful natural and long-lasting colour.
- Fake Bake products give good long-lasting results and there are no parabens or artificial preservatives in them. You can get a professional Fake Bake tanning treatment in spas and salons around the country.
- Xen-Tan is establishing itself as a celebrity favourite and is another long-lasting tan that fades naturally. Their website (see page 280) will help you find a salon in your area offering a professional treatment.

TIP! Instant wash-off tans can be just the thing for a glam summer event. They're a little easier to apply than self-tanners that develop over time as you can see where you're putting them – although you should still follow the same rules to prepare your skin. They're really good for camouflaging minor blemishes and if they have a touch of shimmer, they look great on legs and across the décolletage. Be careful not to apply too much on your face. I apply mine to my brow bone and cheeks for a natural-looking glow. My all-time favourite is Rimmel Sun Shimmer, which comes in six shades and is available in most high-street chemists. Did I mention it's also a total bargain?

Skin-saving body treats

We spend a lot of time worrying about our complexions and often forget to treat the skin on our body to some TLC, particularly in winter when we're wrapped up in layers of clothing. Here are a few treats for your body, which will make you feel lovely, too.

TRY A HOME-MADE BODY SCRUB

I discovered a little home-made recipe that works just as well as any pricey shop-bought exfoliator. All you need is some coarse sea salt and olive oil. Mix them together to form a thick paste, then grab a handful and rub gently over your body to slough away dead skin cells. Pay special attention to your thighs, bottom, the tops of arms and anywhere you have dry, flaky patches, such as knees and elbows. Be careful of any cuts or

TIP! For an extra boost (and wonderful fragrance), add two drops of an essential oil to your home-made olive oil and salt scrub. Try relaxing lavender in the evening or zingy lemongrass for a morning wake-up call. My favourite is rose oil for its anti-ageing properties and gorgeous scent. Note that essential oils shouldn't be used if you're pregnant.

grazes, though, as salt stings! Hop in the shower to wash off and you'll be left with glowing skin from top to toe. It's also a wonderfully invigorating way to start the day.

DON'T DRY OUT IN THE SHOWER!

Many shower gels and soaps contain sodium lauryl/laureth sulphate to produce lather, but this can dry skin and cause irritation. Instead, choose natural, organic soaps that don't have nasty chemicals – your skin will thank you for it. You'll find good brands in your local health store. The Organic Pharmacy has a great range of natural skincare, with wonderful fragrances from essential oils. Or look out for the Dr Organics range, which is great value; you'll find it in Holland & Barrett.

GET BABY-SOFT SKIN

After every shower, slather on loads of nourishing body cream or oil. Yes, it can be a pain when you're in a rush, but your skin will be silky and you'll feel gorgeous. My mum used to swear by a generous application of olive oil after a bath or shower to keep her skin super-soft. Add a couple of drops of your favourite essential oil to smell sweet, too. Lavender is good before bed as it promotes relaxation, rose is soothing and healing, while grapefruit and lemongrass are revitalising.

TRY DIY HYDROTHERAPY

To stimulate blood flow to the skin, bringing much-needed nutrients, start the day with a steamy shower, then just as you're finishing turn the water to cold for a few seconds. Repeat the hot/cold cycle for two minutes. This is definitely one to start the day rather than trying it before bed as it's so stimulating. You'll feel great afterwards, though. Promise!

Hair today…

As we get older we start sprouting hair in all sorts of unwanted places and it gets thicker and darker as well. It usually appears on the face (over the top lip, on the sides of the cheeks, chin and neck). Then there are the legs, forearms, underarms, around the nipples and bikini line – even on the hands and fingers. Oh, and don't forget the big toes! Yep, not nice.

In my first beauty clinic quite a few of my clients were older women and during their facials they'd often ask me to pluck out any odd hairs on their chins, as they couldn't see them without glasses. At the time I just couldn't imagine having hairs appearing from nowhere on my chin and neck! Now, of course, it's a different story. And to make matters worse, these hairs are sometimes half an inch long before you spot them. Don't tell anyone, but I find the best light to find and pluck random hairs is when sitting in the driving seat looking into the rear-view mirror of my car. Remember to park in a discreet spot!

Here's my advice on how to remove unwanted body hair, leaving younger, smoother, sexier skin.

AT HOME

Perfect plucking

For an at-home eyebrow shape, tweezing is still the best option. Make sure you get a good, sharp pair of tweezers – I like Mac's slant-tipped tweezers with texturised tips for extra grab-ability. Take care not to over-pluck your brows as they'll take forever to reappear and if you've been over-plucking for years, they might not come back at all.

Eyebrow replacements

If you've over-plucked your eyebrows so the hairs have stopped growing, you can actually have an eyebrow transplant! Individual hairs are taken from the scalp and transplanted to your brow where they are meticulously angled to follow the desired line of your eyebrow. The hair will fall out within four weeks, but the follicle will have been securely transplanted and within 10 to 12 weeks a new hair will grow permanently. The Wimpole Clinic's Dr Michael May has lots of experience in this field.

If that's not for you, semi-permanent make-up can recreate your eyebrows and will last up to five years. Be careful about the therapist you choose for this, though, as once it's there, it's not easy to remove. See page 281 for contact details for advice on this.

Get fuzz-free with creams

Hair-removal creams have come a long way since the 'one-size fits all' products of yesterday. Now there are spray-on formulas, in-shower creams, bikini-line kits and sensitive skin products. I still think creams are a better DIY option for facial hair than wax strips, which can be tricky to use and a bit messy. Try Nair Sensitive Facial Brush-On.

Sugar, sugar

This is similar to waxing in that you heat the product, apply to skin and remove with cotton strips. I think it's a better DIY treatment than waxing as it leaves less redness, is easier to remove and doesn't have the same pain factor. It's also far less messy as the sugar just melts away leaving skin smooth and soft – there are no nasty globules of left-over wax to contend with. Try The Body Shop Sugaring Hair Removal or Sugar Strip Ease.

Hand-held devices

There are some good hand-held DIY hair-removal gadgets that use pulsed light to permanently get rid of hair. I tested one called Silk'N and thought the results were excellent – and a lot cheaper than going to a clinic for a professional treatment with intense pulsed light. It feels a bit like being pinged lightly with an elastic band. It'll take a few sessions before you start seeing results, but because it's a home treatment you can do it at your leisure. It's good for targeting hair on arms, legs and bikini line.

AT THE SALON

Waxing

This is something most of us have tried and it gets good results – although some find it too painful. The therapist spreads warm wax over the hair to be removed – eyebrows, chin, upper lip, underarms, bikini line or legs – then a strip of cloth or paper is smoothed on to the warm wax and very quickly pulled off, taking the hairs with it. It can bring tears to your eyes, especially around your period when your skin is more sensitive. The danger with too much waxing is that you can get ingrown hairs and, if they become infected, you can end up with horrible spots and the possibility of scarring. Make sure you go to an experienced therapist as it hurts more if it's not done properly. Some wax always seems to get left somewhere no matter who does it, and it can be a pain to remove.

Threading

This technique is a traditional method of hair removal in Asian countries, but you can now find threading bars in some of the larger department stores. It's mostly used for eyebrows and other areas of the face and neck and not generally for body hair.

A thread is literally wound around each hair, which is then pulled out quickly. It can hurt a little, but no worse than waxing or plucking. Eyebrows can be beautifully shaped, leaving a really clean line. There's a real art to this treatment, so look for someone with experience. The best therapists hold the thread in their teeth and hands and nimbly weave away, plucking hairs out rapidly. Once you've tried threading, you may never go back to waxing!

Electrolysis

This treatment is generally used to remove hairs on the face and neck (body parts would take too long). A thin metal probe is inserted into the hair follicle and an electrical current is passed through it, either destroying the cells that grow the hair or causing a chemical imbalance, which again causes the hair to be destroyed. It's common to use a blend of both these methods. I have to be honest and tell you that electrolysis hurts. You can have a topical anaesthetic applied beforehand, but when beauticians do it, they don't usually have access to pain relief. It's also a time-consuming treatment; you may die of boredom before you get rid of that unwanted crop. After a treatment, expect your skin to look red and blotchy. You may need up to 12 sessions to remove stubborn hair. It can leave scarring, too, so again be careful in your choice of therapist.

It's quite an old-fashioned treatment, but it's useful for hard-to-reach areas, such as the inside of the nose and ears or for hairs growing from a mole. It's also good for darker skins that aren't suitable for intense pulsed light treatment (see below). And for people with red, grey, white or blonde hair, electrolysis may be the only answer.

AT THE CLINIC

Intense pulsed light (IPL)

IPL is a permanent method of hair removal, which works by targeting pigment, so it's not as successful on grey or blonde hair, or for those with black or Asian skin. This treatment is not without pain – it feels like an elastic band (quite a large one!) being pinged against your skin. There is a device called Harmony that's mostly painless, but you'll need anything from six to eighteen sessions. It can be effective if you're planning Brazilian bikini line hair removal. Personally, I don't think it's a good idea to have anything permanent done; remember my story about the old lady with her fake Madeleine cake breasts? You might find that Brazilians are not so trendy in a few years' time.

IPL sends high-intensity light beams down each shaft of hair. The light hits the root of the hair and shatters it. If the hair is in the growing stage, the root will be destroyed and that hair won't grow again. However, hair grows in three phases, so there's only a one in three chance that the hair will be destroyed. If the hair root is in the resting phase or about to fall out, you'll have to try again. That's why you need up to 18 sessions.

You can't have a tan when you go for this treatment because the light targets pigment and you could end up with some nasty brown marks that could last up to 18 months. And don't expose your skin to the sun for six weeks after treatment – because the skin has been traumatised, it's more likely to be stimulated by UV light and produce excess pigment, leaving you with brown patches. You also have to grow the hair for a few days before the treatment, so winter is probably the best time. That way you can keep your legs covered up while growing the hair.

TIP! If you have darker skin and are thinking about having IPL, ask for a test patch in a place that won't show, so that if it does mark you will be able to cover it. And be very careful who does this treatment for you as I have seen clients who've been burned by it.

Laser hair removal

Laser hair removal is very popular. It targets the pigment in the hair follicle only, so it can be used on darker skin (although not black skin). This treatment is less likely to burn than IPL but, as with IPL, you mustn't expose your skin to the sun for six weeks before or after the treatment. The results will depend on your skin tone, your hair type, and the growth phase of the hair. You'll need between six and twelve sessions.

As with IPL, you'll be asked to have a few days' worth of hair growth. The practitioner will probably apply a cooling gel, as the laser produces a lot of heat. This will make it more comfortable – although that's probably the wrong word! I won't lie to you. It can hurt, but it's not unbearable.

The duration of the treatment depends on the size of the area being treated. A small area, such as underarms, may take only minutes, while your legs could take up to an hour. Your skin may be red or irritated afterwards, but this will calm down in a day or two. It's important to use sunscreen for six weeks following the procedure, although I'd advise using sunscreen whenever your skin is exposed to UV light. You should also avoid any products that may irritate your skin such as harsh astringents, and don't pluck or wax in the area.

Clinics usually use the term 'semi-permanent' to describe laser hair removal as you may get a few rogue hairs appearing after a couple of years.

Conclusion

Treating your skin well on a daily basis is the key to keeping it in wonderful condition. Great skin is a huge asset and if you put in a little effort and get into a regular beauty routine, you'll reap the rewards with a clear, healthy, hydrated complexion. And well-cared-for skin is the perfect canvas for anti-ageing products and treatments to work on. You'll discover all about these in Chapters 5 and 6.

three
The Beauty of Wellbeing

As I always tell my clients, you can spend all the money in the world on expensive skin creams and rejuvenating treatments, but if you're not taking good care of yourself, it might as well be money down the drain. Lifestyle plays a huge part in how your skin ages, which is why it's important to stay active, get enough sleep, have a healthy diet and not to smoke or drink too much alcohol. Each of these wellbeing elements will keep your skin fresher for longer and ensure you feel great, too.

By looking after your health, you're sending out a message that you like who you are. And being comfortable in your own skin is an important factor in staying youthful. Happiness and confidence are powerful anti-agers. There's nothing more attractive and vital than a beautiful smile.

I think 'all things in moderation' is a great motto for life. There's nothing worse than a food or exercise bore, so aim for a healthy balance. For me this means eating well during the week and having treats at the weekend, getting at least two early nights every week, taking a little time out to de-stress with yoga or a pampering massage, and trying to go for a brisk walk in my lunch hour. It's all about putting yourself first – do that and it'll go a long way to helping you look and feel younger for years to come.

You are what you eat

Beauty is not just skin deep. What you put into your mouth is reflected in your appearance. Eating a balanced diet will ensure your body gets all the nutrients it needs and you'll reap the benefits by enjoying youthfully glossy hair, strong nails and more radiant skin.

So the quest for beauty starts on the inside. Don't expect expensive lotions and potions to stave off the ravages of time unless you're eating plenty of anti-ageing foods.

HOW YOUR DIET PROTECTS YOU FROM AGEING

To keep yourself looking young, your diet needs to be rich in the following:

Antioxidants

These natural anti-agers help fight off the 'free radical' damage that triggers premature ageing. Free radicals are harmful molecules that invade and destroy the cells in our body, and wreak havoc with our skin. They are impossible to avoid as they're a by-product of normal bodily functions, such as breathing, and surround us in the environment. But we can help protect ourselves from their attack by filling our bodies with antioxidants from the food we eat.

The key antioxidants in foods are: vitamins A (found in liver, dairy products, eggs, dark green and yellow fruits and veg), C (fresh fruit and veg, herbs and berries) and E (plant oils, nuts, seeds, eggs, milk and avocados); the minerals copper (found in shellfish, offal and nuts), selenium (Brazil nuts, wholegrain bread and eggs), and zinc (meat, milk and shellfish); and the phytochemicals carotenoids (found in carrots, sweet potato, kale and spinach), flavonoids (apples, berries and red grapes) and phenols (tomatoes, peppers, tea and berries).

For a more detailed list of foods rich in antioxidants, see below.

DID YOU KNOW? Free radicals are produced when we're exposed to external toxins such as cigarette smoke, UV light and air pollution, so it is possible to cut down the number you encounter by not smoking, wearing sunscreen and avoiding heavily polluted areas.

Omega 3 fatty acids

These essential fatty acids reduce skin inflammation and promote skin elasticity and moisture, which helps keep wrinkles at bay. They are vital for healthy cells and help promote blood flow. Without essential fats the skin loses radiance, becomes dry and flaky – and therefore looks older.

Studies have also suggested that fatty acids can increase the chances of survival after a heart attack, reduce the mental decline associated with old age and help prevent changes in the eyes that can lead to blindness.

Foods rich in Omega 3 include oily fish, such as salmon, sardines, mackerel and fresh tuna, along with walnuts, olive oil, pumpkin seeds, soya beans and flaxseeds.

BRILLIANT FOODS TO MAKE YOU BEAUTIFUL

Your anti-ageing diet should include as many of the following superfoods as possible, every day:

- Almonds – they are packed full of protein and Omega 3 fatty acids, which help skin repair itself. They're also a great source of the potent anti-ageing antioxidants vitamin E and selenium.

- Beans – these are rich in free-radical-fighting antioxidants and skin-plumping protein. All beans are beneficial – butter, broad, borlotti, kidney – even the common baked bean, with the tomato sauce providing a dose of antioxidant lycopene.

- Berries – blue, black and red berries and dark cherries get their colour from the antioxidant flavonoid anthocyanin. Studies show this can strengthen the walls of small blood vessels, helping to prevent unsightly thread veins. They also stimulate oil and collagen production to boost the youthful appearance of your skin.

- Brazil nuts – these are the richest natural source of selenium for younger-looking skin.

- Broccoli – this super-veg contains a variety of antioxidant phytochemicals that help stimulate the production of enzymes that detoxify cancer-causing and ageing chemicals in the body. They also improve your skin by stimulating oil production and aiding in the production of collagen.

- Chicken or turkey – both great sources of high-quality low-fat protein, which will help keep your skin elastic and toned.

- Chocolate – oh yes! People who eat it regularly live on average one extra year. This is due to phenols (a type of antioxidant) found in every woman's favourite treat. Dark chocolate contains the most antioxidants so allow yourself a few squares.

- Cucumber – the peel is made of silica, a building block of skin-plumping collagen.

- Eggs – these are excellent sources of the antioxidant zinc, and vitamin D, which is vital in fighting the signs of ageing.

- Brightly coloured fruit and veg – these are all are jam-packed with antioxidant vitamins. The best of the bunch are: kiwis, which contain twice as much vitamin C as oranges; carrots and tomatoes, which are rich in anti-ageing betacarotene; avocados, which are full of healthy fats, iron, potassium, magnesium and vitamins A,

C and E, which rejuvenate the skin and reduce eye puffiness; and apricots (fresh or dried), which are full of lutein, an antioxidant Harvard University scientists discovered helps fight off the ageing effects of the sun.

- Green tea – this contains anti-ageing antioxidants, which is probably why celebrities such as J-Lo, Victoria Beckham and Gwyneth Paltrow are all such devotees.
- Multigrain bread – is packed with the antioxidant selenium. The more seeds it contains the better.
- Oily fish – the Omega 3 essential fats found in salmon, mackerel, fresh tuna steaks and sardines provide skin-loving antioxidants. The high protein content of oily fish also helps keep skin firm – and has the added bonus of keeping you slim. Eat two portions a week.
- Olive oil – a study in the *Journal of the American College of Nutrition* found that people living in hot countries have fewer wrinkles if they have high intakes of olive oil.
- Orange and lemon rind – these are full of broken-vein reducing nutrients called bioflavonoids. Grate it into salads or on top of yoghurt.
- Porridge – studies show that oats contain high levels of a mineral called salicylic acid that plumps up the cells in skin, slowing the appearance of fine lines and wrinkles.
- Probiotics – levels of friendly bacteria in the gut drop significantly after the age of 50, leaving you at increased risk of a sluggish digestion and bloating. Drinking a probiotic drink or eating probiotic yoghurt every day can combat this.
- Prunes – they contain some of the highest levels of antioxidants found in any food.
- Shellfish – they are rich in the antioxidants copper and zinc.
- Soya beans and milk – soya contains isoflavones, plant hormones that are physically identical to the female sex hormone oestradiol.

It helps protect against heart disease and osteoporosis and may ease menopause symptoms. Studies have also shown that soya milk helps speed up the production of collagen. Try swapping your regular milk for soya milk in tea, coffee and on cereal. And snack on soya beans (the Japanese call them edamame beans), which taste great warm or cold, with a little salt or soy sauce.

Your ultimate beauty-boosting menu

Try some of the following ways of eating more anti-ageing superfoods:

Forever-young breakfast
Porridge made with soya milk, topped with a handful of blueberries and almonds. Washed down with a cup of green tea.

Skin-saving smoothie
Simply blend blueberries, pitted cherries and strawberries (a small handful of each), with an avocado, low-fat yoghurt, semi-skimmed milk and a little honey.

Look-lovely lunch
Low-fat cream cheese with red pepper, baby spinach leaves, cucumber and tomatoes on wholemeal bread, followed by a low-fat probiotic raspberry or cherry yoghurt.

Age-delaying dinner
Grilled chicken breast with lemon and almond sauce, served with

tomatoes and broccoli, followed by a fresh fruit salad, which includes cherries, red grapes and kiwi fruit. (To make the chicken, simply squeeze the juice of half a lemon over it, season with salt and pepper and sprinkle with a handful of chopped almonds before grilling for about 25 minutes.)

For a more indulgent version, grill the chicken breast, then, in a saucepan, combine 30g butter, 1tbsp lemon juice and a small onion (finely chopped) and cook over a medium heat. Once the onion has softened, add a handful of chopped almonds and a little parsley and pour over the chicken breast.

Face-saving treat

Dip strawberries into melted dark chocolate for an antioxidant-packed treat. Delicious!

FOODS TO AVOID

Steer clear of the following skin destroyers to keep your complexion as youthful as possible:

- Alcohol – I'm afraid this is the curse of the devil to your skin. It is notoriously dehydrating and causes the small blood vessels to widen, producing flushed skin, broken veins and wrinkles. Ideally, limit it to weekends and try a white wine spritzer, in which the alcohol content is diluted with fizzy mineral water. And remember to drink plenty of still water between alcoholic drinks to avoid dehydration. Your skin and your head will thank you for it the next day!

Supplements for super skin, hair and nails

- Omega 3, 6 and 9 supplements – Omegas 3 and 6 are known as 'essential fatty acids', which means they are necessary for health; however, the body doesn't produce them, so you need to get them from dietary sources or supplements. Omega 9 fatty acids are made by the body, but there's no harm in topping them up. You'll find Omega 3 in oily fish such as salmon and mackerel, and flaxseed oil. For Omega 6, choose sunflower oil, nuts, pumpkin seeds, dairy products, whole-grain bread, eggs and poultry. Good sources of Omega 9 include olive oil, olives, avocados, almonds, peanuts, cashews and sesame oil. I like to take a supplement as it contains the perfect balance of all of these fatty acids, which have great skin-, hair- and nail-boosting qualities. They improve skin from the inside and can also help balance hormone levels.

- CoQ10 – a powerful antioxidant, normally made by the liver, this keeps cells healthy and helps fight free radical damage. From the age of 20 the liver gradually loses its ability to make enough CoQ10, and by the age of 40, our levels have dropped by a quarter. Without enough CoQ10 our energy will drop, leaving us tired and vulnerable to illness. While it's possible to boost your level of CoQ10 through your diet, many women don't enjoy the foods rich in this enzyme – such as heart, kidneys and liver! Rather than forcing myself to eat offal, which I'm not keen on, I find it easier to take a supplement.

- Sugar – this speeds up the breakdown of elastin and collagen in your skin. Try to eat foods with a low glycaemic index (a ranking system for carbohydrates based on their effect on blood glucose levels). That basically means ditching white bread, pasta and rice for wholegrain varieties and steering clear of sweets and puddings.

- Coffee – caffeine stays in your body for up to 12 hours and can mess with your beauty sleep. It's also a natural diuretic so if you drink too much it may have a dehydrating effect on the body – which is not good for your skin. If you love it, go for decaf instead or limit yourself to one cup in the morning. Alternatively, try a herbal tea or make fresh mint tea (simply add a few sprigs of mint to a cup and add hot water).

- Processed foods – ready meals and other fatty convenience foods are packed with nasty additives that can trigger inflammation in the skin and create skin-wrinkling free radicals.

THE FACE/FIGURE DILEMMA

French actress Catherine Deneuve famously once said: 'A 30-year-old woman must choose between her bottom and her face.' What she meant was that as we grow older, striving to maintain a youthfully slim figure can mean sacrificing a youthfully plump face. However, this doesn't mean that you have to let yourself get fat.

Over the years, our metabolism slows down and the amount of lean muscle decreases, which means working harder to stay as slim as we were in our youth. While giving in to middle-age spread is a telltale sign of age, striving to be unnaturally slim is not the way to stay youthful either. In fact, unnatural drastic weight loss can make your face look concave and haggard with very obvious wrinkles.

As you get older the amount of fat in your face naturally reduces. This fat plumps out wrinkles and lips, and makes your pores look smaller as they are supported and don't stretch. If you lose too much fat from the face, you get a hollow look that adds years to your appearance. From your 30s onwards your skin also becomes less elastic so when you lose fat from your face it can become saggy, as it no longer has the elasticity to spring into place.

Over the years, countless women have come to agree with Deneuve's proclamation about a woman's bottom/face dilemma, including many fellow celebrities. I believe there's a balance to be struck, as in all things. Your figure might become a little fuller than it was in your 20s, but so long as you're still a healthy weight, don't fret about it. The main thing is to find your body's natural weight, the one you can maintain easily, and at which you look and feel your best all over.

Say no-no to yo-yo

If I could offer you just one piece of advice, it would be to keep your weight steady and healthy. Don't try any crash diets or drastic exercise regimes. Whenever we lose weight, more fat comes off our face than our body. During crash diets there's no way the ageing skin can spring back after this sudden loss of fat and, what's more, crash diets eat away at the lean muscle that keeps the face firm, causing even more sagging.

Yo-yo dieting, where you get into a cycle of losing weight and then putting it back on, increases your risk of developing many age-related disorders, including the bone-thinning disease osteoporosis. This is because over the years your body doesn't consume enough calcium to ensure healthy stores – so you could find that you have the frail bones of an 80-year-old while you are still only 40. Extreme weight fluctuations also increase your risk of diabetes and heart disease, double your risk of kidney cancer, and can wreak havoc with your fertility.

Can a pill help you stay young?

Nutraceuticals, a combination of the words nutrition and pharmaceuticals, are supplements that have been developed to provide the building blocks the body needs at the optimum levels to provide protection against ageing, with some claiming to reduce wrinkles by up to 30 per cent. However, make sure you pick skin supplements with the right ingredients, such as collagen, ceramides and high strength antioxidants, to be confident they will do what they promise. My favourites are:

- Age Defender by ScioTech, which contains vitamin C and amino acids to fight free radicals and encourage the body's natural production of collagen and Omega 3 essential fatty acids.
- Photo Resist, also by ScioTech, which is a supplement packed with anti-inflammatory properties to help deal with immediate skin damage – take twice a day before, during and after sun exposure.
- Dove Spa Strength Within, which contains lycopene, Omega 3 and vitamins C and E.

Avoid a fitness frenzy

The good news is that you don't need to slog away for hours in the gym to look younger – in fact the opposite is true. Extreme exercise is very ageing. While a bit of exercise is important for health, keeps your muscles toned and gets the blood pumping to the skin, giving you a youthful glow, too much intense exercise can make you look haggard.

But how much is too much? Experts say running more than 10 miles a week or doing other high-impact exercise (such as aerobics, step classes or tennis) for more than two hours a week is excessive.

In the 1980s, a New York-based cosmetic surgeon coined the phrase 'jogger's jaw' to describe the premature ageing caused by exercise and weight loss. If you watch a runner in slow motion, you can see the tissues of their face moving up and down. This movement stretches and lengthens the collagen and elastin fibres of their skin, which reduces skin tone and helps contribute to sagging jowls and cheeks.

Rather than over-exercising, I suggest you find ways to include moderate exercise in your daily routine. Could you walk to the shops rather than driving? Do you have time for a quick workout at lunchtime? Or why not take the kids on a bike ride or for a kick about at the weekend?

Here are a few more easy ways to sneak in some exercise:

- Put on your favourite music and dance around your living room (while nobody is around, of course). You can burn 100 calories in just 15 minutes. You could also try a workout DVD or, if you fancy being more sociable, join a salsa or ballroom class.
- No time to exercise? If you have only five minutes to spare, climb those stairs instead of taking the lift. You'll burn between 100 and 150 calories if you do it quickly, and it's a great cardiovascular workout.
- Nominate two evenings a week when you don't use the TV remote to change channels. Just getting up and down a few times over the course of an evening can burn extra calories. Squatting down when you switch channels is also a good workout for your legs and bum.
- Shop till you drop. Pounding the high street with heavy bags will help you burn calories and tone arms, but make sure the bags are well balanced to avoid over-exerting one side.

- Dusting, cleaning, vacuuming and scrubbing are as good at fighting flab as a gym workout. Cleaning windows for 30 minutes burns 250 calories, washing the car 330 and ironing for an hour 210. In comparison, 10 minutes on an exercise bike pedalling at 70rpm sees off only 60 calories. For optimum results, hold your tummy muscles in as you clean. This is a great multi-tasking tip for busy women!

- A little bit of bedroom fun can do wonders for your waistline. Research shows that the average sex session burns 150 calories per half-hour, increases your heart rate, improves circulation and reduces stress. When you make love you use many parts of your body and your breathing and heart rate increase, which is equivalent to – and can be even better than – pounding the treadmill. As well as the fat-burning bonus, regular sex will also flood your brain with feelgood chemicals called endorphins that increase your happiness level.

- Gardening is a great way to get some peaceful 'me time' and just think of the sense of achievement you'll feel if you manage to grow your own salad or veg. Even tidying, trimming and pruning can be hugely rewarding. And it'll burn calories, too, without you even noticing – up to 350 calories in one hour if you're doing physically demanding activities like mowing the lawn.

Sleeping beauty

A good night's sleep is one of the most important things you need to look fresh-faced and youthful. If you don't get enough, those wrinkles will appear deeper, circles darker and your complexion duller – as I discovered to my own cost recently. I had some photos developed of a night out with friends and when I saw them I was horrified! Once I'd calmed down, I remembered I'd had a terrible sleep the night before, which explained the dark circles, sallow skin and slightly haunted look. I'm sure that had I got my usual eight hours I'd have looked much younger.

Most of us need between seven and nine hours of sleep a night to feel great, but trying to stay on top of all the stresses of modern life – work deadlines, housework and demanding kids – means that getting our beauty sleep quota can seem like an impossible luxury.

Here's how to improve the quality and quantity of your shut-eye:

- Create a sleep haven. Keep your bedroom quiet, dark and comfortable. The ideal room temperature for sleep is moderate to cool – too hot will hamper your ability to drop off. Even the slightest noise or light can disturb sleep, including the ticking of a clock or the standby light on your laptop or TV. If necessary, use earplugs and blackout curtains to ensure you sleep through the night.
- Ditch the extra pillows. While a headboard covered in pillows might look inviting, it won't help you fall asleep. Being more or less perfectly horizontal is conducive to many of the physical changes associated with slipping into a deep sleep. Throw all but one pillow off the bed.
- Chill out! Schedule in a relaxation period and stop doing anything that's stressful or requires concentration 30 minutes before bedtime. The best sleep-inducing activities are the boring ones. If you have trouble sleeping, you need to find an activity that takes your mind off trying to get to sleep, but at the same time is dull enough not to stimulate the brain too much. When it comes to bedtime stories, put down that thrilling page-turner and re-read an old favourite.
- Pass on the coffee. That cup of coffee at lunchtime could be the reason you're still up at midnight. If you have had too much caffeine, try a cup of chamomile tea, which has a sedative effect.

Or try eating a small snack containing carbohydrates, which have a naturally soporific effect. A study at Sydney University found that eating carbs before bed could boost tryptophan and serotonin, two brain chemicals involved in sleep.

- Lower the lights. A couple of hours before you're planning to go to bed, dim the lights in whatever room you are in. Use soft sidelights instead of the harsh overhead one. This will remind your body clock what time of day it is and it will start to wind down.

- Quit smoking. Apart from all the other terrible side effects, having a smoke before bed puts a stimulant into your bloodstream, which has a similar effect to caffeine. Nicotine can keep you up and make you more likely to wake in the night. The best thing is to quit, but if you're a determined smoker, try not to have one for at least two hours before bedtime.

- Try not to clock watch. Don't have any clocks facing your bed or you'll be tempted to keep checking the time and figuring out how many hours you have left before you need to get up. Your mind will start to dwell on this and it will keep you awake longer.

- Banish booze. Alcohol may initially help you to fall asleep, but as your body clears it from your system, it can cause symptoms that disturb sleep, such as nightmares, sweats, and headaches.

- Have a good soak. A bedtime routine is not only important for children. Getting into the habit of having a relaxing bath before bed will give you time to unwind and switch off from your stress-filled day. It will also soothe and relax your body, relieving it of any niggling aches that could keep you awake.

- Have a liquid curfew. Try not to drink anything too close to bedtime, or you run the risk of waking in the night because you need the toilet.

- Stick worries on ice. We've all experienced that horrible feeling where you lie in bed but can't sleep because all your problems are running through your mind. Put negative thoughts to bed by writing them down, then put your list of worries in a different room and remind yourself that there is nothing you can do about them at this moment and that you'll be better able to deal with them after a good night's sleep.

- Eat right, sleep tight. It's not a good idea to go to bed on an empty stomach but it's also wise to avoid heavy meals close to bedtime, as they can cause indigestion or acid reflux, in which the contents of the stomach travel back up the oesophagus. If you can't avoid a late-night meal, doctors advise you sleep on your left side. This is because your stomach is on the left side of the body, and the oesophagus enters it from the right. Lying on your left means the oesophagus is higher than your stomach, keeping the stomach contents away from it and preventing reflux.
- If your body is pleasantly fatigued from exercise you will sleep better. But if you get too energised or become more alert after exercise, it's best not to exercise after 7pm and switch to morning or lunchtime workouts instead.
- Listening to soft soothing music can give your brain something to focus on rather than the fact you can't sleep. Many stereos have a sleep function whereby they turn themselves off after a set time, and there are even CDs designed for sending you to sleep. Some are just gentle classical music, while others have the sound of waves or a drumming rhythm that mimics a heartbeat.
- Another way to stop your thoughts keeping you awake is to tune your radio to a channel that is continuous talking (no music) such as Radio 4. Turn it down low, so that you have to concentrate hard to make out most of the words. Focus on trying to follow what is being said and you will gradually drift off to sleep.
- Avoid napping in the day or having lie-ins at the weekends if you're prone to insomnia, as this will disrupt your internal body clock and make it hard for you to drop off the following night.

Snacks to help you sleep

The right snack, containing compounds that have a relaxing effect on the brain, can be the perfect sleep inducer. Scientists believe that these natural sedatives work by stimulating the brain to produce calming chemicals, which promote a feeling of drowsiness. If you have trouble dropping off to sleep, eat one of these snooze-inducing snacks 40 minutes to an hour before bedtime for a good night's rest:

Honey with oatcakes
Simply spread two oatcakes with plenty of pure honey.

Honey is soporific because of its high sugar content. It boosts serotonin levels and induces feelings of tranquillity, which should help you drop off. The oatcakes are full of carbohydrate, which stimulates the body to produce more of the hormone responsible for making us feel sleepy after a meal. They're also low in calories!

Fresh strawberry and pineapple smoothie
Chop and hull ten strawberries and chop two large slices of fresh pineapple. Blend with 250ml of semi-skimmed milk.

Milk contains natural opiates called 'casomorphins' that have the power to make you feel drowsy. Pineapple contains bromelide, an enzyme that aids digestion, which means food won't lie in your stomach and stop you sleeping. Strawberries simply add tons of flavour – plus loads of beauty benefits, as they're such a good source of skin-boosting phytonutrients and antioxidant vitamins.

- Forget sheep! Research at Oxford University found that people instructed to think about a relaxing scene before trying to sleep were more likely to drop off than those asked to count sheep.

- Avoid eating, watching TV or discussing emotional issues in bed, as you may end up associating the bed with these distracting activities and that could make it difficult for you to fall asleep. Keep your bed for sleeping and sex.

- Still struggling to sleep? The worst thing you can do is lie there fretting about how little sleep you're getting. It will just make matters worse. Trust that you will sleep eventually and in the meantime just relax and breathe slowly. If you can't get to sleep for more than 30 minutes and are starting to fidget, get out of bed and do something boring in dim light – like filling in your tax form. That should send you off in no time!

And relax

Stress makes you look old and haggard, and predisposes you to all sorts of diseases. It keeps you awake at night, and ruins the quality of your sleep. In fact, stress is one of the single most debilitating things for your skin, body and spirits.

I hate the way stress makes you feel and I hate what it does to your body. As far as I'm concerned, stress is Public Enemy Number Two when it comes to your skin – second only to sun in the damage it can cause. So you need to bin it – and fast.

Whenever I feel stressed, I give myself a good talking to. My favourite mantra is: 'If stress did any good, it would be useful; but as it doesn't, then ditch it!'

Of course, there is no way to protect yourself entirely from stress. All of us, no matter what our job or family situation, will experience stress over the years, so the key is to find effective ways to tackle it and minimise the damage when it does comes along.

Here's my advice on combating the day-to-day strains:

- Make a list. Often we feel stressed because it seems we have so much to do that it would be impossible to get it all done in one lifetime. When you're feeling swamped, sit down and write a list of what you need to do. Include everything from the most important thing to trivial matters you're worried you'll forget about. Then work out which things are the most urgent and start ticking them off the list. When you break your workload down into bite-sized chunks, it won't have the power to overwhelm you.

- Pack away your troubles. At the end of every day, look at what's left on your 'to do' list. Resolve to get as much as possible done tomorrow and then put it all out of your mind until then.

- Get up and moving. It's easy to slump on the sofa when you're stressed, but this will make you feel worse. Instead take a brisk walk. The endorphins your body naturally produces when you exercise make you feel good, and ease stress. Physical activity plays a key role in reducing and preventing the physical effects of stress, so factor in some yoga or swimming twice a week.

- Think positive. Stop dwelling on the past or worrying about what the future holds. Visualise good things happening to help you think more positively and stop stressing.

- Never soldier on alone. Talking through any problems with your partner, a trusted friend, GP or even a counsellor can help lift the burden.

- Slower-paced music can lower your heart rate and blood pressure. I find listening to a bit of soothing classical music can work wonders at reducing my stress levels.

- Schedule time to breathe. Set the alarm in your mobile phone to ring in five minutes, find a quiet place (even if it's in the toilets at work) and just sit there breathing slowly and deeply, in and out, until you feel calmness wash over you.

- Laughing temporarily increases your heart rate and blood pressure, and then when they drop afterwards, you feel instantly more relaxed. Watch your favourite sitcom or funny movie, and give in to the giggles.

- Restrictive clothes (especially those that put pressure on your stomach) cause your muscles to tighten, which in turn makes you tense. As soon as you get home lose the skinny jeans and stifling shirt and throw on some comfy PJs.

- Set aside specific times to be alone and do absolutely nothing – well, nothing important anyway. This is time for you to enjoy, so watch a favourite TV programme, flick through a celeb magazine, have a bath or go for a stroll – whatever you feel like. The important thing is that you turn off your phone and don't let work or other commitments encroach on this time. If you have kids, finding the time to do nothing isn't easy, so negotiate with your partner for a few precious child-free hours. It'll help you recharge your batteries and allow you space to just be you. I think having a bit of time off makes you a better mum, too, so don't feel guilty!

- Many people find that a hobby with no deadlines or pressures, which can be picked up or left easily, takes the mind off stresses. This probably explains the recent knitting craze among female celebs and why many people love a good crossword or Sudoku.

- Learn to say 'no'. Taking on more than you can handle is a sure-fire recipe for stress. Whether in your personal or professional life, know your limits and stick to them. When you're close to reaching them, refuse to accept added responsibilities. It might be hard at first, but you'll be glad you did it.

- Give yourself enough time. Being late for work, nursery, the school run or social events will mean you're stressed and flustered before you've even arrived. Always allow extra travel time before any event and you'll be able to swan in smiling and relaxed.

- Look for the good. Try to view stressful situations from a more positive perspective. Rather than getting annoyed when you're stuck in traffic, look at it as an opportunity to pause and enjoy some alone time or listen to the radio.

- Accept you're not perfect. Striving for perfection is a major source of avoidable stress. Stop setting yourself up for failure by demanding that you are a super employee/mum/wife/daughter. We're all human, we all get things wrong sometimes, so don't beat yourself up.

- Stick to your healthy diet. It can be easy to resort to comforting junk food when the pressure is on, but well-nourished bodies are better able to cope with stress, so watch what you eat.

- Avoid sugar slumps. The temporary buzz you get when eating sugar ends with a crash in mood and energy. If you reduce the amount of sugar in your diet, you'll feel more relaxed and you'll sleep better.

- Learn to meditate. Studies show that meditation helps us to manage our reactions to stress effectively and to recover more quickly from disturbing events. It allows your body to rest and stress hormones to subside, and it occupies your mind so that unpleasant or anxious thoughts don't intrude. I think regular meditators and yoga fans actually look younger, too, as they don't seem to have that permanently worried frown.

My simple meditation

Sit in a comfortable chair with your eyes closed and think about a place you find relaxing, such as a beautiful beach or garden. Once there, focus on your 'in' breath and imagine it lifting from the base of your spine to the top. Then imagine your 'out' breath flowing back the other way. Try to keep your mind free of other thoughts as you relax and picture the place you've chosen. 'Walk around' it, 'feeling' the soft sand or cool grass beneath your bare feet and the warmth of the sun on your body, and 'listen' to the soothing sounds of the waves lapping the shore or the bird song from the trees. Get lost in your special place, imagining all the sights and sounds until you feel ready to come back to reality.

TIP! If you find it hard to relax into a meditation, try lighting a candle in a dimly lit room. Watching it flicker can help you get into the right state of mind.

• Treat yourself. Women often feel guilty about pampering them-selves, but I'm telling you now – don't! Regular treats, whether it's a relaxing massage, a night out with friends or simply a luxurious hot bubble bath, can help keep stress at bay and a smile on your face. You're worth it!

Three instant de-stressors

- Mix equal drops of lavender and chamomile essential oils into warm running water for a relaxing aromatherapy bath.
- Try Bach's Rescue Remedy. Many people swear by this blend of natural flower extracts. Just a few drops on the tongue can promote a sense of calm.
- Do a DIY tension relief massage. Place your thumbs on your cheekbones close to your ears, and use your fingertips to gently apply pressure and rub the temples. Then, using very firm pressure and a tiny circular motion, gradually move your fingers up along your hairline until they meet in the middle of your forehead, massaging your entire forehead and scalp as you inch along.

The happiness factor

Like most women, I'd like to be a bit thinner, less wrinkly and to lose the double chin, but I can fix those things if I really want to. In the meantime, I can honestly say I love my life. For me there's nothing better than dinner in a nice restaurant (with pudding and cheese), a glass of champagne, seeing my friends for a natter or staying up late sometimes. I've never been as happy as I am now, and I really wouldn't turn back the clock. I have a wonderful family and a great job. Yes, I have more wrinkles than I did 20 years ago, but I can count my blessings.

Women are never more beautiful and vital than when they're happy. Here are a few ways to find happiness and ensure that contented glow shows on your face:

- Have more sex. Making love three times a week can boost your mood and make you look 10 years younger, according to recent Scottish research. A vigorous sex life was found to be one of the most important factors in how young a person looked.

- Try acting happy and confident, even if you're not feeling it. Just as applying your favourite lippy can make a difference to your mood, the first step to feeling in a better mood is to start acting happy – even if you're feeling down. If you add extra zing to the way you come across, people will respond to you more positively – and that in turn will make you feel better about yourself.

- Don't make comparisons that will only make you miserable. In particular, don't compare yourself with the celebrities you see in magazines; they all get airbrushed to death, so what you see is not reality.

- If you ever find yourself feeling bad about your life or the way you look, use this quick strategy: remember a time when you felt really confident in your appearance, then take a deep breath and as you let it out, let yourself feel good.

- Keep smiling. A smile is worth a million dollars in beauty terms. A positive expression will not just make you feel good about yourself; it will also knock off several years. Studies show that smiling faces are always perceived as more youthful than sad ones. Plus, smiling is infectious. If you smile at someone, they'll smile back, boosting the feel-good factor all round.

- Make an effort to look good every day and you'll feel instantly more attractive. Blow-drying your hair, applying a touch of make-up and picking out your most stylish and brightly coloured clothes doesn't cost a penny.

- Don't forget to compliment others. Make an effort to tell friends and colleagues how great they look, especially when they've made an effort or seem a bit down. It'll make you feel great when you see how much of a boost you've given them and, just like smiling, compliments are infectious, so you're sure to receive a few in return.

Conclusion

When it comes to making lifestyle changes, please don't feel daunted. Lots of small, easy tweaks can make a huge difference to how you age. Whether it's making a conscious effort to find a little more 'me' time, building more activity into your day, getting to bed earlier a couple of nights a week or swapping a few naughty nibbles for a handful of nuts – it all adds up.

I've found that when you start making a few changes and begin to look and feel better as a result, it spurs you to keep going. You won't want to trade in that glowing skin and happier outlook for those old, familiar habits. You'll like the 'new you' too much.

four
Simple Tricks to Turn Back Time

Recently I found myself looking at an American website called 'Not Your Daughter's Jeans', which sells jeans that flatter less-than-perfect figures. Being the mum of a gorgeous 17-year-old girl who's 5ft 10ins tall with a figure to die for, I thought, 'Um, sounds interesting!' I'd love to be able to wear jeans like my daughter Sophie, but I'm 5ft 3ins and a size 12 on a good day.

When I stumbled across the website I thought I'd struck gold and ordered three pairs immediately. The best bit is, you can order a size smaller than you really are – how's that for a feelgood boost? They have a tummy tuck panel (perfect for new mums), your muffin top stays nicely in place, your tummy looks washboard flat, they're comfortable beyond belief and you don't look like mutton dressed as lamb. What's not to love? When they arrived I ran them past Sophie, who assured me they looked 'great'. And this from the girl who cries 'No, Mum!' every time I pick up an item to try on in Miss Selfridge.

The point of this story is that we can wear most things as we get older – we just need to adapt them a little. And the same is true when it comes to updating our hair and make-up. Trust me, there's a very happy balance to be found between a twinset and pearls and squeezing your wobbly bits into the latest wetlook leggings. You only have to look at all the women currently in their 40s, 50s and beyond who look gorgeous, hip and sexy – and there's not a dodgy cardigan or string of pearls among them. Think Michelle Pfeiffer, Halle Berry, Jennifer Aniston, Demi Moore, Sarah Jessica Parker, Christie Brinkley, Iman, Julia Roberts, Elizabeth Hurley. The list goes on! OK, you could argue they have plenty of cash to spend on beauticians and stylists – but we can all have access to the same beauty products, treatments and insider advice.

Take it from one who's been in this business for a long time, with access to the latest and greatest cutting-edge treatments: there's a lot you can do yourself to look younger for longer without spending a fortune or going anywhere near a Botox needle. Some clever hair, beauty and fashion tricks can go a long, long way.

Here are my no-fail ways to drop a decade, without trying too hard.

Nothing adds ten years like … bad hair

Women get comfortable with their hairstyle – so comfortable they don't change it for decades – but an outdated style adds years to your look. If you still have an 80s perm or your streaky blonde do is more Princess Di than Kim Cattrall, it's time to make a change.

As you age, you need to soften your colour and alter the length. Too short is harsh and unforgiving, while too long is inappropriately girly. Likewise, if you're in your 30s and sporting a hairstyle that wouldn't look odd on your grandmother, you need to loosen up. Here's how to get it right.

DROP A DECADE

Get rid of greys

Some women go grey gracefully and look fantastic. Actress Helen Mirren, for example, still looks sexy even when she lets her hair go its natural silvery grey. How does she do that? But for most of us mere mortals, grey hair is incredibly ageing and I'm a big believer in covering it up as soon as the first strands appear, which for most women is around their early to mid 30s. If you only have a few greys you don't need to have an all-over colour. Instead, go for a few lowlights or highlights that blend in with your natural shade. If you have a lot of grey, you'll need a permanent colour all over, but go for a shade that's lighter than your own hair so the greys don't look too obvious when they start coming through. Adding some subtle highlights will also soften the look. A good product for covering up greys between salon visits is Clairol Root Touch-Up, a permanent dye that gets rid of grey roots in around 10 minutes.

> **TIP!** If you have a grey roots emergency and you're brunette, use a little black or brown mascara to cover them up. Make sure you don't overload the brush, then apply it to your parting and blend in gently with your fingertip. Old mascaras that have dried out slightly work best, so don't throw them out!

Get the colour right

Jet black, fiery red and white blonde are too harsh as we get older because our skin tone becomes paler. To avoid looking washed out, the trick is to lighten dark shades, go for auburn instead of bright red and warm up blonde shades with honey tones. A solid block colour can also be too harsh. Ask your hairdresser to add highlights or lowlights to break it up, giving you a more natural look.

If you're black or Asian, jet black will look natural, but any greys will really stand out, so you'll have to dye your hair regularly to keep them covered up.

> **TIP!** Lightening your eyebrows a little will soften your face – and blend in any stray greys. You could try this yourself by applying a little facial hair bleach, but take care when using the product close to your eyes and leave it on for just a minute as it'll work fast. If you're not confident enough to attempt this yourself, ask at your local beauty salon.

Get the right length

When I was on holiday 25 years ago, I saw a very slim woman with long raven hair wearing a bikini on the beach. When she turned round, instead of being in her early 30s as I'd expected, she was at least 55. It was horrible, and the memory still sticks in my mind today! If you like long hair, cut it to shoulder length. It's much more flattering and still long enough to look good if you put it up or curl it.

Hair that's too short is also a big no-no as it'll show up any double chins or drooping jowls on the horizon. A little length will soften your features and draw the focus away from imperfections. In my view, pixie crops are best left to teens and 20-somethings.

Enjoy fringe benefits

Fringes can hide a multitude of sins – such as forehead wrinkles and frown lines. Soften the look by having your fringe feathered to take away some of the volume. A side-swept fringe is also very flattering.

Don't overdo your do!

However old you are, a look that's too 'done' is old-fashioned and incredibly ageing, so that means no big hair, backcombing or stiff hair-sprayed styles. If it's more volume you're looking for, try oversized heated rollers for a lift at the root and a soft curl. You can also get more volume when you're blow-drying by using a volumising mousse and a large round brush. Lift sections of your hair towards the ceiling and blast the roots with heat. There are lots of thickening or volumising shampoos and conditioners – just remember to apply conditioner only to the ends of your hair.

TIP! If you must use hairspray, avoid stiff, sticky hair by applying the spray to your hands first then smoothing it over. Or spritz the hairspray into the air and walk through it. Much more subtle.

The tousled look

If you have longer hair, try this styling tip for a tousled, just-out-of-bed look with plenty of body. Blow dry your hair so it's nearly dry then divide into about eight sections. Take each section and twist it round into a sausage, then pin it on to your head in a circle shape. Leave for 20 or 30 minutes while you do your make-up, then unpin it. Shake it out, apply a light serum for extra shine and definition, and *voilà* – soft, sexy waves with almost no effort at all!

Try a sexy up-do

A scraped-back ballerina bun can be harsh and super-ageing. Instead, go for a looser topknot, allowing strands at the front to fall around your face – so much more flattering.

Let it shine

Nothing screams youth and vitality more than super-shiny hair. As we get older, hair becomes drier and loses its lustre. Try taking a supplement containing Omega 3, 6 and 9 fatty acids, which are great for hair health. Once every two weeks, use a hot-oil treatment from the chemist or an intensive hair-conditioning mask. And when you're at the hairdresser, accept a free head massage if they offer one – this will boost blood circulation to your scalp.

TIP! For a DIY hot oil treatment, boil some water in a pan, then take it off the heat and place a glass bottle of olive oil in it. Once the oil has warmed up, drizzle it on to your hands and smooth it through washed, towel-dried hair. You don't need to apply it to the roots. Wrap your hair in a towel or shower cap and relax for 30 minutes. Afterwards, jump in the shower and rinse your hair with warm water, then give it a light shampoo.

Love your layers

Have a few layers cut in – this will give your hair bounce and body, which it loses as you get older, and it'll soften your face, too.

Maintain your style

Try to have a trim and get your colour done every six weeks to help maintain the condition and avoid straggly split ends.

Nothing adds ten years like … bad make-up

Make-up from another decade is a dead giveaway when it comes to revealing your age. Frosted lipstick, too-blue eyeshadow, overdone blusher and foundation three shades darker than your skin say only one thing to me: 'I learnt how to put on make-up circa 1985.'

It's not just being stuck in a make-up rut that can age you. Too much make-up isn't a good look on anyone, whether you're 25 or 55. Trowelling on thick foundation is the worst sin of all as it 'deadens' your complexion, making it look dull and flat instead of youthful and radiant. When it comes to your base, you want it to look as though you're barely wearing any make-up at all but still look fabulous. Good make-up should enhance your natural beauty, emphasise your best features and minimise flaws, while allowing your skin's natural glow to shine through. It should never be painted on like a mask.

Here are my golden rules for younger-looking make-up that really will take years off your face.

DROP A DECADE

Use a primer

Many women still don't apply a primer before their foundation because they're not really sure what it's for. So here's the story! Primers even skin tone, minimise fine lines and pores, and cover imperfections to create a smooth base for your foundation and help it to last longer. Make-up artists swear by Laura Mercier Foundation Primer. Some primers include brightening ingredients to give your complexion extra radiance.

Brighten up

In the past couple of years, skin-brightening products have become popular. They're also known as face highlighters, illuminators or complexion enhancers. The idea is that they bring your skin alive, giving it a natural-looking glow, which is perfect for more mature skin because we lose that luminosity as we get older. You can wear it on bare skin if yours is good enough, under foundation or you can spot-apply it to cheekbones and brow bone as a highlighter. I like Clinique Up-Lighting Liquid Illuminator and Benefit High Beam.

Get your foundation right

As we age, foundation becomes more important than ever to help even skin tone and cover flaws and blemishes. The trick is to avoid heavy matte foundations, which settle in wrinkles making them look deeper. That 'caked' look won't let your skin's natural radiance shine through. Remember, less is more!

Choose lighter hydrating formulas that help plump out lines instead of emphasising them. Foundations with light-reflecting pigments give skin a youthful luminescence – or try mixing a little illuminating primer with your regular foundation.

Most modern foundations provide good coverage without looking obvious and 'cakey'. Some, such as Max Factor Colour Adapt foundation, even adapt to your skin tone for a really natural match.

If you have good skin that's relatively flaw-free (lucky you!), a tinted moisturiser may be all you need as a base for daytime. It won't give you the same coverage as a foundation, but it'll look more natural and won't highlight fine lines. I like Chantecaille Just Skin Anti-Smog Tinted Moisturiser SPF 15 and Laura Mercier Tinted Moisturiser SPF 20.

My tips for flawless foundation

Give your moisturiser a few minutes to sink in before applying your make-up. This will help foundation stay put and it'll go on more smoothly.

For the best finish, apply a primer before your foundation to minimise all those little blemishes and imperfections, and provide a really good base. It should also mean you'll need less foundation, so you'll get a more natural look. I prefer to apply it just to the T-zone where there are open pores.

Apply foundation with clean fingertips or a sponge if you prefer. Only use it where you need it. Take it just below your jawline but not halfway down your neck, where it can mark your collar. If you've got the right colour, it should blend in seamlessly.

Apply a light-reflecting wand concealer such as YSL Touche Éclat under your eyes to reduce dark shadows and blend in with your ring finger. Cover any blemishes with a thicker cream concealer.

You should now have the perfect canvas on which to apply your blusher and eye make-up.

I'm not wild about loose powder on top of foundation – probably because I remember my granny's thick, slightly orange powder compact, which contained talc so it settled in lines and wrinkles making them much more obvious. Modern powders, however, are lighter and cleverer. If you like to use some to set your foundation and minimise shine, go for a translucent one with light-reflecting pigments that don't flatten your complexion. Dust lightly over your face, avoiding any lines around your eyes or mouth.

Finding the perfect colour match

To find the perfect shade of foundation – which should be as close as possible to your natural skin colour – try it on your jawline instead of the back of your hand. And make sure you take a mirror compact when you hit the shops so you can check out the colour in daylight before you buy. I like to apply it to half my face to see how it suits my skin.

Ask for samples at beauty counters or take in your own small containers and ask for a few squirts of the tester products so you can try them at home. Foundation can be a pricey purchase these days, so it's worth taking a little time and effort to find the perfect one before you part with your cash. If you want to take the legwork out of it, go for Prescriptives Custom Blend, where a consultant mixes a shade to suit your complexion perfectly and a record is kept for future orders.

In this country it used to be almost impossible to find good foundations for women of colour, but I'm glad to say that many of the big cosmetic houses now have ranges that suit black, Asian, Middle Eastern and Hispanic complexions and hopefully the choice will continue to improve. Try Maybelline, Bobbi Brown, Mac, Prescriptives and Clinique. Gorgeous Somali-born supermodel Iman has a make-up range, Iman Cosmetics, which she developed out of frustration at never being able to find the right shade for her own skin.

Try switching to mineral make-up

I'm a huge fan of mineral make-up and much prefer it to traditional liquid foundations. I use mineral make-up every day and I also apply it on clients who are going back to work or to an event after having a facial as it doesn't penetrate the skin. They are always amazed by the results and walk out feeling a million dollars.

It gives fantastic coverage and the most flawless finish of any make-up I've tried. This means it's perfect for more mature skin and skin that needs a little extra help to cover problems such as age spots, scarring or rosacea and it works well on skin with acne, too. It also contains those all-important light-reflecting pigments to reduce the appearance of fine lines.

Mineral make-up is a lot easier to apply than liquid foundation. It comes in a compact and you simply sweep it over your face with a large brush. You don't need to use a lot to get good coverage, so it lasts for ages and is great value for money.

My advice is to go for a pressed powder version rather than a loose powder, which can leave a 'powdery' look on your face. Loose powder is also harder to apply and blend in, and can be messy.

Mineral make-up uses naturally occurring minerals – titanium dioxide, zinc oxide and iron oxide – which are purified and crushed into fine powder. It naturally provides broad-spectrum sun protection and contains no nasty chemicals or oil, so has virtually no allergy risk and won't block pores. Beware of any brands that include talc in the ingredients, though, as this causes the powder to float and settle in wrinkles.

Applying mineral make-up

For very natural-looking coverage with mineral foundations, the best brush to use is a luscious kabuki brush, which has a short rounded head. If you want light coverage, go for a brush with long, loose hair. For maximum coverage, you'll need a denser short-hair brush. A powder dome brush is good on dark or black skin, which needs a few light applications rather than one heavier one.

Brushes that use real animal hair are the best and my favourite brand is Brush Up. These brushes use the best first-cut hair (from the tips of the fur), which is super-soft and cruelty free.

It's important to keep your brush clean as it can harbour bacteria. Clean it by massaging in a little shampoo and rinse under tepid water till it runs clear. Leave the brush standing upright to dry. Never leave it soaking in water as this could damage the glue and cause the hairs to fall out.

To apply mineral make-up with your chosen brush, start on your forehead and work the powder into your skin in small circular motions, going all over your face including your eyelids, lips and beneath your jawline. Once you've applied the foundation, stroke the brush down your face to get rid of any excess powder and to make sure any downy hairs are lying flat.

You can use a good mineral make-up on your eyelids to protect the delicate skin from the sun. If I'm out and about somewhere hot, I also put a light dusting on my ears, neck and décolletage to prevent sun damage.

Because good mineral make-up is made using only skin-healthy ingredients, the products are interchangeable and can be used anywhere on the face – for example, a blusher can be used as an eyeshadow or even as a lipstick mixed with a little gloss. My favourite brand of mineral make-up is Mineral Earth.

TIP! If you're stuck in a make-up rut and don't know how to get out of it, have your make-up done professionally then recreate the look at home. Most beauty counters in big department stores offer a make-up makeover and will offset the cost against any products you buy. Just remember to be clear about the look you're after and make sure they take into account your age and skin type. Or take a make-up lesson; you're never too old to learn new tricks and it'll be money well spent.

Get a rosy glow

As we get older, cream blushes are best, as powders can emphasise fine lines and make mature skin appear dry instead of dewy. It's said that the perfect blusher should make you look like you've just finished a workout or had really good sex!

Apply a couple of dots of cream blush to the apples of your cheeks and blend in and outwards towards your temples so there are no obvious lines. Use a small amount at first – you can always build up the colour if you need to.

Fair skin suits pale pinks, medium skin looks good with peaches and rosy pinks, while brown tones and corals suit dark skins.

TIP! In summer, try bronzer instead of blusher. The trick is to apply it only where the sun would naturally hit – on your cheekbones, brow bone and collarbone – for a naturally sun-kissed look. Never apply bronzer all over your face and neck; it looks fake and overdone.

Soften your eyes

Say goodbye to black eyeliner, ladies! Once you hit 40, tons of rock-chick black liner is far too harsh. Greys and browns are much more flattering and you'll still get a nice smokey effect. If you're applying pencil under your eyes, make sure you soften the line by smudging it a little to avoid that hard 'drawn on' look. Or use a flat liner brush and apply a little shadow under your eyes instead of pencil.

Avoid bright blue, green and purple eyeshadows at all costs – unless you want to look as though you've just been made up for the West End stage!

TIP! To brighten eyes instantly and make them look wide awake, run a white or nude pencil along the eye rim. This opens up your eyes and is much more flattering and modern than using black or blue liner inside the eye.

Bat your lashes

As we age, our eyelashes become more sparse so it could be time to add a volumising mascara to your beauty must-haves. There are plenty to choose from and you don't have to spend a fortune to get a good one, although some of the cheaper ones can clog lashes. I like Max Factor False Lash Effect Mascara and Benefit Bad Gal Lash.

Dyeing your lashes is another way of making them appear thicker and longer. Even if you have dark lashes they will be fair at the ends, so dyeing them makes a difference. Try a home dye such as Eylure 45 Day Mascara Eyelash And Brow Dye Kit, or get them professionally dyed at your local beauty salon. It's not an expensive treatment and you'll love the results. It's a great idea before a summer holiday – just think, no more rivers of mascara running down your face after a dip in the pool!

You could also give false lashes a go. They can be fiddly to apply yourself, but once you get the hang of it the effect is fantastic. Groups of single lashes can give a natural result and look great when applied just to the outer corners of your upper lids.

> **TIP!** Falsies aren't practical for every day, so if it's something more permanent you're after, check out the latest trend for eyelash extensions. This is a beauty salon treatment in which each false lash is bonded to one of your own, making your lashes look naturally fuller and longer. They last for between four and six weeks and you can get away without wearing any mascara at all. A perfect low-maintenance look!

Go for shimmer, not glitter

We all like to inject a bit of glamour into our make-up for a night out, but beware of glitter. Unless you're a teen or 20-something, it's just too over-the-top. That glittery eyeshadow Lily Allen wears so well will crack at the first sign of a wrinkle. That doesn't mean you can't shine, though. Go for a less obvious approach with creamy satin eyeshadows that have a slight sheen or shimmer. Use lipgloss with a little sparkle as a topcoat over your lipstick, and apply some face highlighter to your cheekbones and brow bone. Subtle, but super-sexy!

TIP! Emphasise your eyes or your lips, but never both. If you're going for dramatic smokey eyes for a night out, keep your lipstick neutral. If you'd like to wear a vampy darker shade of lipstick, keep your eye make-up subtle.

Perfect your pout

As we get older, the rule with lipstick is to avoid anything too dark, too light or too bright. Dark reds and plums make lips look smaller and meaner, and it's more obvious when they bleed into those vertical lip lines. The same goes for bright tomato red or orange, and anything too pale can make you look washed out. Pinks and neutral shades are super-flattering and give the illusion of plumper lips. Go for hydrating lipsticks or glosses and apply a nude lipliner first (as close to your natural lip colour as possible) to define your mouth and help prevent bleed.

TIP! Get your mouth ready for lipstick with a super-quick exfoliation. Simply rub your toothbrush over your lips after you've brushed your teeth to get rid of flakiness. Next, apply a little lip balm and leave for a few minutes before putting on your lipstick. This will banish dryness and help it glide on smoothly.

Nothing adds ten years like ... bad teeth

Recently, research found that discoloured teeth can make you look not ten, but 13 years older. That doesn't surprise me at all. The fact is, as we age, teeth naturally darken and years of drinking tea, coffee and red wine, smoking and eating dark-coloured foods lead to stains. But in my opinion there's no point in making an effort to keep your hair, skin and clothes youthful, if you then open your mouth to smile and reveal a row of yellow teeth – not sexy! The good news is, there are things you can do to get a whiter, brighter, more youthful smile. Here's how.

DROP A DECADE

Have a whitening treatment

Having your teeth professionally whitened by a dentist can achieve great results. The treatment lasts around 90 minutes and involves applying a bleaching agent to your teeth, which is then activated with a light or laser beam. Most dentists will also send you home with custom-made trays that fit your teeth exactly, along with whitening gel so you can carry on with the whitening at home. I've found this treatment a little painful, although lots of people don't find it uncomfortable at all. You'll be more prone to pain if you have sensitive teeth.

Three easy ways to whiter teeth

- Avoid lipsticks with brown, coral and orange tones as these tend to make your teeth look yellow. Deeper pink and red tones will make them appear brighter.
- Avoid wearing bright white next to your face as your teeth will look discoloured in comparison.
- For a DIY whitener, put a little toothpaste on your brush, then top with some baking soda and brush normally. Don't do this every day, though, as baking soda is quite abrasive.

If you want to bleach your teeth, my advice is always to have it done professionally rather than buy a DIY whitening kit from your chemist. The bleaching gel in these kits is very weak, and the trays won't fit snugly to your teeth, so the gel can leak on to your gums and cause pain.

TIP! Replace mercury fillings with white ones before you have a whitening treatment so you get a good colour match.

Get a Hollywood smile

If you weren't lucky enough to be born with a smile to rival that of Julia Roberts you can buy one – but it doesn't come cheap. Porcelain veneers – wafer-thin coverings that are bonded to the surface of your teeth – can radically improve your smile, but they could end up costing thousands if you need several. The good news is that veneers last for 20 years and you won't need to bother with whitening treatments. They're really strong and look natural, too. They're a good choice if your teeth are crooked, uneven, short, gappy or worn down rather than just discoloured.

Nothing adds ten years like ... bad nails

We pay attention to the skin on our hands, using creams and sun protection to avoid age spots and crêpey skin, yet most of us barely give our nails a second thought. But let me share a little secret, ladies – nails age, too! As we get older, ridges start to appear, nails become drier and break more easily, and they can take on a nasty yellow discolouration. Nobody wants 'old lady nails', so here's how to get them in tip-top condition.

DROP A DECADE

Smooth the bumps

Ridges are like wrinkles for the nails; they look horrible and we get more of them as we get older. They're easy to smooth by sanding the surface with a nail buffer. Only do this once a week, though, to avoid nails becoming thin and more prone to splitting. You can also buy nail treatments to target the problem, which you can wear alone or as a base coat under your regular nail polish. Try Opi Ridge Filler, Mavala Ridge Filler or, for a bargain buy, check out Revlon Nail Support Ridge Filler Base Coat.

Avoid the splits

Our nails become drier and more brittle, but with a little care you can stop them splitting. Go for a gentle, moisturising nail polish remover that doesn't contain acetone, as this is harsh on nails and dries them out even more. You should also wear cotton-lined rubber gloves if your hands are in and out of water a lot.

There are plenty of cuticle creams on the market designed to nourish cuticles and promote stronger, healthier nails. A nice one is Burt's Bees Lemon Butter Cuticle Cream, which uses natural ingredients including lemon oil and it smells great, too. However, I don't believe you have to buy a separate cuticle cream if you don't want to – your regular hand cream will do just as well. Just make sure you spend a little time massaging it into your cuticles. Alternatively, for a no-frills cuticle treatment that works really well, use olive oil from your kitchen cupboard.

There are clear nail-hardening polishes with nylon fibres that help to strengthen nails, which you can use alone or under your regular varnish. Always have a couple of polish-free days a week to allow your nails to breathe.

Get a younger shape

Long, pointy talons are definitely not hip! They look witchy and dated, particularly when they're painted fire-engine red. Modern nails are short (no longer than just past the end of your finger) and squared off, with the corners gently rounded. I've heard the desired shape called a 'squoval' and I think this describes what you're after perfectly. This shape will keep nails healthier and less prone to splitting. The length is also perfect for all nail shades from nudes right through to dark plums.

Fix the colour

Discoloured nails aren't pretty! Buffing them can help get rid of discolouration but, to cover them up, go for baby pink, sheer white or pale pastel polish to cancel out yellow tones. Dark reds and plums, which are very on-trend right now, will cover any nasty discolouration completely.

> **TIP!** Don't forget your toenails. They might not be on show all the time but they need just as much TLC, so follow all the same rules. When trimming toenails, cut them straight across with clippers and file gently, taking care not to file the corners down as this could lead to ingrown nails.

For more on de-ageing your hands, see pages 209–15. For more on foot-care, see pages 251–5.

Nothing adds ten years like ... bad clothes

Remember when you were in your teens and 20s? Practically your entire life was dedicated to fashion (along with make-up, music and boys). If you were anything like me, you knew all the latest trends and which celebs were wearing them, and where to find the best bargains on the high street.

As we get older, it's easy to lose touch with fashion. Our lives become taken up with kids, jobs and running the house, and we just don't have the time to keep up to date with every new style or spend hours window-shopping on a Saturday afternoon.

Luckily for me, my daughter Sophie is a fount of fashion knowledge and a good sounding board, but if you haven't got a Sophie at home, start buying fashion magazines. There are several on the market aimed at women over 30 and most have websites, too. Another tip is to check out celebrities who are a similar age to yourself and steal their style. What are they wearing when they take the kids to the park and how do they glam up for the red carpet?

Wearing last season's trends or, even worse, last decade's trends will instantly age you. We all have those items we can't bear to part with: that pair of stretchy jeans, those comfy shoes. And most of us have wardrobes crammed with clothes we bought years ago that we hardly wear but can't bring ourselves to part with. Take my advice: if you haven't worn something in the past year, you're not going to. It's time to get ruthless! Have a big clear out and deposit anything that makes you look old and doesn't flatter your figure at the local charity shop. If you need some advice, rope in your sister or a best friend who will tell it to you straight. Trust me – you'll feel liberated and ready to revamp your look. Here's how.

DROP A DECADE – OFF-DUTY CHIC

Be a jean genius!

When it comes to jeans, unless you're a super-trendy teen or 20-something, avoid skinny-leg, ripped and bleached styles. Low-rise jeans, which are cut super-low on your hips, aren't a good idea either as even the tiniest of muffin tops will bulge over the top! Likewise, high-waisted styles might hold in your tummy but they'll make your bum look huge unless you're very slim. For me, the perfect pair of jeans is dark blue denim (very slimming) and boot cut. The slight flare balances out bigger thighs and looks great with heels to make legs look longer. If you prefer a slimmer leg go for a straight cut and make sure the waistband sits just above your hips to help hold in any wobbly bits.

Dress to impress

Dresses are an easy option. Go for simple, block-colour shift dresses, wrap dresses, anything tailored and styles which nip you in at the waist. Avoid anything that swamps your figure, such as big bold prints or empire-line styles that make you look pregnant. Tea dresses with ditsy prints are a good option and also look good in winter with opaque tights. Add a little dark denim or leather jacket for a great off-duty look or team with a blazer for a smarter take on this trend.

Don't skirt the issue

In my opinion, once you hit 35, micro-minis and minis should get the boot. Even if you're a size zero, those knees will be starting to get slightly crêpey. Even with thick tights, short skirts can look a little 'mutton'. Go for a hemline that sits an inch or so above the knee or on the knee. Hemlines that fall below the knee or sit mid-calf are old-fashioned and ageing and, unless you're tall, will make you look as though you're standing in a hole!

Buy a Little Black Blazer

This should be a wardrobe staple. Dress it down with jeans, heels and some statement jewellery for a laid-back night out or team with a pretty dress and ballet pumps. In fact, this classic piece goes with just about anything.

> **TIP!** You only need to invest in a couple of key pieces such as a blazer or a dress each season to update your wardrobe. Or use accessories to stay on-trend – a scarf, bag, a pair of shoes or some costume jewellery can revamp existing outfits without costing the earth.

Don't go figure-hugging all over

Supermodel Elle Macpherson may look amazing in tiny, super-tight bandage dresses well into her 40s but, for most of us, a really clingy outfit will just show up a multitude of sins and can look tacky. A good rule is to go tight on the top or bottom half, but never both. So if you're going for a close-fitting top, team it with wide-leg trousers or a looser-fitting skirt. If you're wearing slim-leg jeans or a pencil skirt, go for something with more volume on top such as a silk tee or blouse.

Watch the fabric

Any clingy synthetic fabric rings alarm bells with me – it literally shows up every lump, bump and bra bulge. Not attractive! Save Lycra for the gym and choose natural fabrics that hang nicely on your curves rather than looking sprayed on.

Dress for your shape

If you have a bigger bottom and thighs, go for darker block colours on your bottom half and choose wide-leg or boot-cut trousers with a flat front and broad waistband. Opt for A-line skirts, which flare out nicely over your hips and thighs.

If you're trying to deflect attention from a bigger bust, avoid busy prints and choose V-necks instead of tops with a high neck. Avoid fussy scarves draped over your boobs, as this will just draw the eye to the area. Go for nicely fitted tops – you don't want to look matronly – but make sure they're not clingy.

If flabby upper arms are your bugbear, look for three-quarter-length sleeves. Cap sleeves are a big no-no. If you want to wear a sleeveless dress or top, just team it with a cute cardie.

For big tummies, go for looser-fitting dresses and tops that will skim over the problem area. Think silk tees and blouses worn loose over jeans. A long-line tunic top with slim-leg jeans is a great weekend look and is perfect for hiding big bottoms as well as wobbly tums.

Get fancy with your footwear

Shelve the sensible shoes and opt for something a little sexier. Heels make legs look slimmer and longer, and I think they make you feel great, too. I wouldn't advise skyscraper platform stilettos, but take your heel a little higher and see what it does for your legs. Thicker heels are more comfortable and stable than skinny stilettos.

Fitted knee-length leather boots (flat or with a heel) are really flattering and look great with opaque tights and a skirt, as well as over slim-fitting jeans.

Leave trainers for the gym. If it's comfort you're after, go for ballet flats, simple lace-up canvas pumps or wedges with a low heel. They all look great with jeans.

DROP A DECADE – AT THE OFFICE

Makeover your suit

I think skirt and trouser suits are dull, old-fashioned and ageing. Go for chic separates instead. Try a cropped, swing or Chanel-style jacket with a pair of classic black wide-leg trousers and heels. Team with a fine-knit sweater, plain tee or fitted shirt and accessorise with a few long strands of beads.

A sharp pencil skirt with heels and a blouse is another good look. For summer I like to wear a slim white skirt with a black short-sleeved blouse and some killer courts – it's a classic look that never dates.

Dresses are another easy look for the office – team with a little black blazer, a cute cardie or try belting a smart long-line cardigan over the top.

Avoid 'old lady' tights

Flesh-coloured tights like your granny used to wear are a complete no-no. Remember that fetching orange shade of American Tan? Avoid that like the plague!

For winter, choose opaque tights in black, brown, navy and grey – much more 'now' and very slimming. In summer, go for bare legs and nude heels (always closed toe for the office). Don't forget to make sure your legs are hair-free, well-moisturised and nicely tanned (fake, of course).

Smarten up your bag

A leather shopper or oversized tote are the perfect work bags: smart, on-trend and big enough to carry everything from magazines and

> **TIP!** When it comes to younger-looking accessories, don't forget your glasses. A pair of granny glasses will do nothing for your specs appeal, particularly if you have to wear them a lot. Spend some time at the optician's experimenting with different styles. Thinking 'style' instead of 'practicality' is a good starting point. And don't be afraid to ask the sales assistants for help. They're usually pretty good at helping you work out which ones suit your face shape best.

newspapers to your laptop and desk diary. Tatty briefcases, satchels and rucksacks must go!

DROP A DECADE – NIGHT-TIME GLAMOUR

Shrug off bingo wings

I see women of all ages at my clinic who hate their saggy or flabby upper arms. But as we get older the problem gets worse due to a combination of loss of muscle tone, cellulite and crêpey skin. Luckily, there are loads of good options for covering them up so you still get to wear your strappy cocktail dress. Go for shrugs, pashminas, bolero jackets, smart cardies with three-quarter-length sleeves and little sheer or lace jackets. Look for the special occasion or wedding floor in big department stores or try shops such as Coast and Monsoon, which do occasion wear.

Say yes to Spanx

Find some good figure-fixing underwear to slim, smooth and boost in all the right places. Celebs have been wearing Spanx pants underneath their red carpet frocks for years to keep their bums and tums under control. Shapewear (as it's referred to) is big business and much prettier than it used to be. There is literally an undergarment for every problem: a slimming slip to smooth your silhouette under a close-fitting dress; cycling shorts to control a wobbly bottom and thighs; and waist-cinchers and briefs that will give a flat mum bum a lift. Check out the lingerie section of big department stores or the website www.figleaves.com. Marks & Spencer has a body-sculpting underwear range called Magic.

Invest in a Little Black Dress

Every woman – whatever age she is – should have one of these in her wardrobe. The LBD is classic, slimming and you can change the look and dress it up or down using different accessories.

Use statement jewellery

An oversized statement necklace is perfect to update a simple dress and it'll help to cover crêpey skin, too. Swap a single string of pearls (very 'old lady') for long strands of pearls, beads and chains. Wear a few clashing strands together for a look that's really 'now'. Stacks of bangles are also a hot look that you don't have to be 25 to wear.

Dress down

These days, unless you're going to a ball or a wedding, you can get away with a less formal look for a night out. Try jeans or wide-leg trousers with heels, a silk top, a cute jacket or blazer and loads of fab jewellery.

Save the bling for your accessories

Sequinned, metallic and neon outfits scream 'Look at me!' and I think they're best left to nightclubbers in their 20s. Personally, I'd feel like a Quality Street wrapper in a gold or silver dress. Save the sparkle for your jewellery or a gorgeous embellished clutch bag. Or choose one piece with a subtle sparkle: try a cardie or scarf with a gold or silver thread running through it or a few sequins.

Beware of plunging necklines (and low-cut backs)

Deep plunging V necks and scoop necks will emphasise crêpey skin, saggy boobs and breast fold lines. Remember what your mum used to say: you don't have to put everything on display to look sexy. Go for a square-cut or round neck if your décolletage is less than smooth and plump. You can still make the most of your bust with a slim-fitting dress or top.

Even if you're super-slim, the skin on your back starts to sag as you get older, so check yours out in the mirror before opting for a backless dress.

> **TIP!** If you're wearing strappy sandals or peep toes, make sure you have perfectly groomed feet and polished nails. Bumpy, discoloured nails are a dead giveaway. Short nails painted with deep reds and plums or nude shades look great. For more on fabulous feet, see pages 251–4.

DROP A DECADE – AT THE BEACH

Be wary of bikinis

Once gravity gets to work on your body, thongs, string bikinis and bandeau tops should be avoided. Even if you're really slim, an itsy-bitsy bikini is unforgiving and you won't get away with even the smallest area of saggy skin. Choose a top with proper support for your bust that has wider straps or a halter neck and underwiring for a lift. Go for a brief that's fuller (make sure the legs aren't cut too high) or 'boyfriend' style pants. Tankinis are a good option for covering stretchmarks or a mummy tummy.

Say yes to a sexy one-piece

Swimsuits are back on-trend (thank God!) and there are loads of really flattering styles around. A one-piece will hold in all your wobbly bits and is much more slimming than a bikini. Cut-out styles are chic and perfect if you have a slim waist – although watch the tan lines if you catch the sun.

There are also some great figure-fixing swimsuits around that sculpt your body and hold you in. Check out the Miraclesuit swimwear range (you'll find it in bigger department stores and from online stockists).

Choose cool cover-ups

Never go on holiday without a couple of chic beach cover-ups. Go for knee-length kaftans and beach dresses – and pack a couple of sarongs, too. These don't take up a lot of space in your suitcase but are really practical. You can tie them in a dozen different ways to hide your least favourite bits. Tie them in a halter, wrap around your waist or wear bandeau style.

TIP! Fake tan makes you look instantly slimmer and will give you more confidence to bare your body on the beach. Get a salon tan the day before you go on holiday so you have an even all-over colour. And never, ever forget your sunscreen, a wide-brimmed hat and sunglasses! For more on faking it, see pages 45-8.

five

The Truth About Miracle Creams

Buying a face cream can be totally baffling. There are literally hundreds of products lining the shelves, all promising to make us look years younger, and which are 'clinically proven' to do this and 'scientifically proven' to do that. The days when you'd pop to your local chemist for a pot of cold cream are well and truly gone.

I recently took my mum to a big department store where she examined the many anti-ageing creams on display and wanted to buy them all. Everything sounded wonderful: 'Face-lift in a jar', 'Eye bag remover', 'Nine minute bottom lift'.

As much as I'd love to tell you there are 'miracle creams' that will have a dramatic impact on wrinkles and sagging skin, there's no such thing. No cream on this earth will give you a face-lift or remove eye bags that have taken decades to form. If it's an instant fix you're looking for, the only way you'll achieve it is with treatments such as fillers and muscle-relaxing injections to ease lines or lasers and peels that change the structure of the skin and have long-lasting effects.

The good news is that creams can do a lot to improve the condition of your skin. They can plump up the surface layer to smooth fine lines, boost radiance and make it feel nice. But you have to be realistic. You're not going to go to bed and wake up the next morning looking ten years younger. Despite what the packaging may claim, there is no such thing as a 'face-lift in a jar'! And you have to persevere. You need to use a cream religiously twice a day for at least a month before you will start seeing results.

I honestly believe you don't have to spend a lot of money on an anti-ageing cream. It's the ingredients that make a product worth buying, and what matters is the percentage of these ingredients in the cream.

It's simple to work this out, as the label will have a descending scale of ingredients. If the one you want appears second or third on the list that's great, but if you find it right down at the bottom, forget it and keep looking.

In my view there are actually only seven key ingredients you need to worry about when choosing anti-ageing products. They may not work miracles, but they do work. Here's what they are and how they can improve your skin:

- Coenzyme Q10 – this powerful antioxidant, also known as CoQ10, speeds up cell repair and aids healing. It's particularly beneficial for menopausal skin. It's worth taking a CoQ10 supplement, too.
- Hyaluronic acid – this sounds scary because of the word 'acid' but it's found naturally in the deeper layers of the skin and keeps it smooth and plump due to its ability to hold up to 1,000 times its weight in water. It's a great choice for mature and dehydrated skin. A lot of the big cosmetic houses are now putting this in their creams. It's also used as an injectable filler to temporarily plump out lines – you'll find out more about this on pages 134–5 and 155.
- Retinol – I love this ingredient. It's derived from antioxidant vitamin A and rejuvenates the skin by boosting cell and collagen production.

DID YOU KNOW? A stronger relation to retinol, Retin-A, is available on prescription only and is often given to people with very thick, sun-damaged skin or acne as it makes your skin turn over rapidly and reduces oil production. A huge part of anti-ageing is about getting rid of those surface layers of dead skin. As we age, skin cell turnover becomes sluggish and that's why we lose our glow and wrinkles look deeper. Retin-A shouldn't be used often, though, because it's so strong. If you overuse it, your skin can become red, shiny, dry and flaky. Not a good look!

- Glycolic acid – I'm a big fan of this ingredient, which can now be found in many high street creams, serums and exfoliation products. Even Boots has products that include it, such as its Time Delay Anti-ageing Gentle Glycolic Peel Kit.

  It's a fruit acid that comes from sugar cane. Fruit acids are collectively known as AHAs (or alpha hydroxy acids), so look out for these on product packaging. Glycolic acid is a brilliant exfoliator, removing dead skin and boosting cell renewal for a luminous complexion. It also stimulates collagen with regular, long-term use.

  I'd recommend using a cream containing it every other day for a week, then every day after that. You must wear an SPF 15+ with it, though, to protect the newer skin from the sun.

  One of my favourite clinic treatments is a gentle glycolic acid chemical peel, which gives great results. Find out more about this on page 136.

- Pentapeptides – these amino acids are small enough to penetrate the epidermis (the outer layer of your skin), stimulating collagen production and helping to keep wrinkles at bay. Palmitoyl pentapeptide (commonly called Matrixyl) is one to look out for.

All *you* need to know about peptides

Peptides are chains of fewer than 50 amino acids and occur naturally in the body, although the ones used in skincare are synthetic. A monopeptide contains one molecule, a dipeptide contains two molecules, a pentapeptide (my favourite) contains five molecules and a hexapeptide contains six. They are the key to turning on cells, and different cells are unlocked by different peptides. For example, hexapeptide 3 will block the enzyme that makes muscles contract, giving a similar effect to Botox. On the other hand, pentapeptides are the key to stimulating collagen.

Here are the main peptides used in skincare products:

- Hexapeptides – these are the muscle-inhibiting ones, so are great for relaxing wrinkles.
- Pentapeptides – as I've mentioned, these increase collagen so are great for plumping and thickening ageing skin.
- Palmitoyl oligopeptide – this increases collagen and hyaluronic acid production so is fantastic for hydration and skin plumping.
- Copper peptide – the copper is delivered to the deeper layers of the skin, accelerating collagen production. It's also an antioxidant so helps with free radical damage and healing.

- Vitamin C – this powerful antioxidant intercepts skin cell damage, boosting collagen production and counteracting sun damage. It also has an anti-inflammatory effect. On the packaging it'll be listed as a derivative of ascorbic acid, such as ascorbyl glucosamine, ascorbyl glucoside, ascorbyl methylsilanol pectinate and ascorbyl palmitate.

- Vitamin E – another super-antioxidant, vitamin E is vital to protect skin cells from UV light, pollution, cigarette smoke, and other factors that produce cell-damaging free radicals. It also increases the effectiveness of sunscreens.

TIP! We all love the sound of a collagen cream, don't we? Collagen is a protein that gives skin its firmness but, as we age, it breaks down and the result is lines and wrinkles. But – sorry to disappoint you, ladies – collagen can't be absorbed through the skin as the molecule is too large. It'll sit on the surface to help lock in moisture and make skin feel nice, but that's it. So please don't buy ridiculously expensive skin creams that contain it and claim to work miracles on wrinkles – they won't!

Miracle creams de-jargoned

I often visit the beauty counters of big department stores but the problem I find is that every salesgirl gets commission on what she sells. When you talk to them about your skin and its needs, you often get really bad advice because they're just desperate to sell you something ... anything! I've lost count of the times I've been recommended products more suited to teenage skin, which I clearly wouldn't benefit from.

But without any alternative guidance it's easy to be lured into buying a product by an advert on the telly in which a naturally gorgeous (and usually very young) supermodel recommends it, or because of its posh packaging and impressive-sounding 'scientific' claims. Remember, it may look fancy and it may sound fancy, but it might not do you any good.

Cosmeceuticals: when you want something stronger

You've probably heard the term cosmeceutical bandied about by beauty editors. It's a term that's been coined to describe products that are a cross between a cosmetic and a pharmaceutical because they contain a higher concentration of active ingredients such as AHAs and retinol than creams you can buy over the counter.

They're mostly available from skin clinics and salons where staff are qualified to assess your skin and recommend these higher-strength products, although you can now buy them from some bigger pharmacies and you'll find certain ranges online. I think it's best to get advice from an expert before making a purchase for two reasons: firstly, to limit the risk of any skin reactions and, secondly, to help you find the right products for your skin's needs – most of these creams don't come cheap!

My favourite cosmeceutical brands are NeoStrata, Jan Marini and MD Formulations.

So what do you do? My tip is to visit a skin clinic or beauty salon at least once and talk to a therapist who has proper knowledge of skin and can give you independent advice. In the long run, it'll save you money because you won't be splashing out on products in the hope you'll stumble across one that works for you.

In the meantime, here's my guide to what you can and can't expect from those 'miracle' anti-agers. I've personally road-tested every product on the following pages and have chosen them based on the ingredients and the results.

Working down the body, from eye creams to cellulite products, I'll share my tips on the best high-street buys that won't break the bank, through to mid-price products and luxury creams that are worth spending your hard-earned cash on. On pages 277–80 you'll find websites through which you can buy them – and all the other products mentioned in the book.

EYE CREAMS

Tired, puffy eyes, crow's feet and dark circles – there's nothing like that little lot to add ten years to your face! Eye creams won't get rid of suitcases under your eyes or banish big black circles, but they can smooth fine lines, boost hydration and tighten skin. The most effective ones include vitamin A in the form of retinol, vitamins C and E, green tea and Coenzyme Q10.

My verdict: always choose a super-light formula or a gel as thick creams can make your eyes even puffier and, when applying it, tap a small amount around the orbital bone (don't take it right up under your bottom lashes). I don't actually think it's necessary to have a separate eye cream if your day cream is light and easily absorbed.

My best buys

- **High street:** Nivea Visage Anti-Wrinkle Q10 Plus Eye Cream
  This includes one of my favourite ingredients, Coenzyme Q10, to help skin cells regenerate – and it's great value, too.
- **Mid price:** Avon Anew Rejuvenate 24 Hour Eye Moisturiser
  This is a real find as most eye creams don't include a sunscreen. This one has broad spectrum UVA/UVB SPF 25.
- **High end:** Clinique Repairwear Intensive Eye Cream Complex
  This includes retinol to boost skin turnover and peptides to help plump out wrinkles.

LIP PLUMPERS

Sadly, these aren't going to give you Scarlett Johansson's super-sexy pout, but the best ones will temporarily plump up your lips. Some give an instant bee-stung look with ingredients such as cinnamon, which irritates your lips and causes swelling in the tissue. Others use ingredients such as dipalmitoyl hydroxyproline (a plant-derived acid) and the peptide palmitoyl oligopeptide to stimulate collagen and boost hydration, so are best used regularly over time to get good results. You'll often find vitamin B12 in the ingredients list, too. This is very nourishing and helps give lips a younger, fuller appearance.

Plumpers usually come as balms, clear glosses and tinted glosses.
My verdict: good for adding a bit of drama to your make-up for a night out or used regularly as part of your beauty routine for smoother slightly plumper lips over time.

My best buys

- **High street:** Maxi Lip Plump
  I really like this bargain buy. It's a glossy balm containing the patented MAXI-LIP™ formula, which stimulates collagen production. And, as it's such fantastic value, you can afford to be generous with it.
- **Mid price:** Freeze 24/7 Age-less Plumper & Gloss
  You can wear this as a gloss over your usual lipstick or alone to enhance your natural lip colour and give a good plumping effect. It's very glossy, so a good one for night-time glamour.
- **High end:** Jan Marini C-ESTA® Lips
  This is one of my favourite anti-ageing brands. It not only plumps but also smoothes lip lines, helping to prevent that nasty lipstick bleed. A good choice for more mature skin. You can see results almost immediately.

DAY CREAMS

Daytime is the most dangerous time for your skin, as it's constantly under attack from ageing UV rays from the sun – whether it's the hottest day of the year or the rainiest. So with this in mind, the most important cream you can put on your face has to be a day cream with an SPF of at least 15. It should provide moisture all day long (there's nothing worse than that taut, dry feeling), and should include antioxidant vitamins C and E for extra protection.

My verdict: always choose a light formula that's easily absorbed, as this will help your make-up stay put. I've tried creams that literally peel off like dead skin if you run your finger along the jawline. Yuck! And remember, it doesn't matter if your cream has a long list of fancy anti-ageing ingredients; if it doesn't have a sunscreen, it's pointless. An SPF is the most important anti-ageing ingredient of all.

My best buys

- **High street:** Olay Total Effects
  As well as being a moisturiser it has a touch of sunless tanner, a gentle exfoliator, a brightening ingredient and SPF 15. It can be a little heavy for some people, but it's worth a try because it literally does everything in one go. Perfect for time-starved women!
- **Mid price:** Harley Street Skin All Day Moisture
  I developed this for myself because I could never find a moisturiser that would keep my very dry cheeks hydrated all day. It has peptides in it, AHAs, antioxidants and, of course, sunscreen.
- **High end:** NeoStrata Daytime Smoothing Cream with SPF 15
  This lovely anti-ageing moisturiser includes glycolic acid and broad-spectrum UVA/UVB sun protection. I love it!

Are there any creams that have the same effect as Botox?

Q: I'm starting to see lines appear around my eyes and on my forehead. I don't want to have Botox just yet. Are there any 'miracle' creams that would give me the same effect?

A: There are creams that can relax wrinkles to a degree. They usually come in the form of serums, so they're lightweight and easily absorbed. The most commonly used ingredient is Argireline, which is the peptide acetyl hexapeptide-3. It works by affecting the enzyme that makes your muscles work. It's nowhere near as powerful as Botulinum toxin A, but it can have a noticeable effect on fine lines and you should see a difference after three weeks of regular use. The effects will disappear, though, within 24 hours of not using it.

Try Medik8 Pretox 20, a muscle-relaxing gel that you use morning and evening, and Harley Street Skin Line Eraser, which I developed at my clinic with needle-phobic women in mind!

NIGHT CREAMS

While we sleep our bodies are repairing some of the damage that's been done during the day. A good night cream should have vitamin C, which stimulates collagen. Other ingredients commonly used in night creams are CoQ10 to aid cell repair, peptides to reduce wrinkles and boost firmness, and AHAs.

My verdict: find a cream that's light so it's absorbed into your skin – you want it on your face, not on the pillow! If you have oily or combination skin, just apply it to areas where you need it, such as your cheeks and neck, otherwise greasy T-zones can get greasier and pores can get blocked. You should also avoid skin oils as these sink into pores, combine with dead skin cells and block pores.

My best buys

- **High street:** Neutrogena Visibly Firm Night Cream
  This is a good budget-friendly cream with copper peptides to improve elasticity and firmness. It's nice and light, too, so easily absorbed.
- **High street:** Avon Hydrofirming Night Cream
  This is a fabulous cream with hyaluronic acid, which is good for dry skin with a lack of firmness. Avon has some good anti-ageing products at affordable prices.
- **High end:** Jan Marini TransFormation Cream
  A light cream that contains transforming growth factors to repair damaged skin cells, as well as vitamin C, hyaluronic acid and retinol. The only trouble with this high-end cream is that if you buy it once, you may get hooked!

DID YOU KNOW? Cosmeceutical companies are increasingly using hormones called transforming growth factors (TGFs) in their creams to stimulate collagen and healing. In fact, we use them in our own Harley Street Skin Stem Cellutions Serum. They were originally used by doctors to heal surgical wounds as they help reduce inflammation (therefore reducing scar tissue) and stimulate cellular healing. TGFs are produced naturally in the body (although the ones used in skincare are synthetic), but as we age they start to decrease, affecting our ability to repair genetic damage, leading to, among other things, lines and wrinkles.

Do I really need different creams for day and night?

Q: Is it essential to buy different day and night creams or can I use one good anti-ageing moisturiser, which I can apply in the morning and before going to bed?

A: I don't believe you need to buy two creams if you don't want to. For some reason, people think it must be better to use thicker creams at night, but these just sit on top of your skin and do no good. If you go for a night cream, make sure it's a light formula such as a serum, so it can penetrate.

If your skin reacts well to your day cream, then use it at night. If it has an SPF in it, don't worry because it won't do you any harm. However, if you want your moisturiser to multi-task for day and night, it's probably best to buy an anti-ageing cream without sunscreen and use it with a sun protection product such as Clinique's City Block Sheer Face Protector SPF 25 or a foundation that includes sunscreen during the daytime. Alternatively, my preference would always be to use a mineral make-up, which naturally contains an SPF of around 20 (see page 91).

INSTANT COMPLEXION BOOSTERS

We all get days when we look in the mirror and think, 'I need help – right now!' Whether your dull, lifeless skin is the result of partying, poor sleep or being kept up for nights on end with a new baby, instant complexion boosters are designed to come to the rescue. They typically contain radiance-boosting vitamins and botanical extracts.

My verdict: instant serums are just that – you get a short-lived effect. If you have the cash to spend on an instant fix like this, go for it, but I think it's a luxury buy. In my view it's better to use products with antioxidants and peptides that will have a cumulative effect to improve the quality of your skin long-term. But if you can afford a complexion booster, it's great to keep in the cupboard for 'off days'.

My best buys

- **High street:** Olay Total Effects Mask
  I really like the Total Effects range – it's a good high-street buy. This product always gets good reviews and it certainly gave my skin a nice healthy glow. As well as having a brightening effect, it hydrates skin and is a gentle exfoliator, too.
- **High street:** Revlon Skinlights Face Illuminator Lotion
  Make-up artists love this product for its fast results. It has light-reflective qualities as it contains particles of rose quartz, topaz and mother-of-pearl, so the light literally bounces off your skin, making you look instantly more radiant and younger!
- **Mid price:** Clarins Beauty Flash Balm
  This is the most famous complexion booster and consistently gets rave reviews in beauty mag surveys. The operative word is 'flash', as you get an instant result so it's the perfect pick-me-up before a night out. It includes radiance-boosting vitamins and is good for all skin types.

LINE 'FILLER' CREAMS

These creams are designed to fill lines around the eyes and mouth temporarily. They typically contain hyaluronic acid, antioxidant vitamins and peptides to plump out wrinkles.

My verdict: most of these ridge fillers are OK for a quick fix to make lines appear softer, but the effect doesn't last long.

My best buys

- **Mid price:** Cosmedicine Instant Wrinkle Write Off Line Filler
  This topical wrinkle filler and line smoother comes in an easy-to-use twist pen and dries in seconds. You can use it over make-up, so you can touch up those lines even when you're out.
- **Mid price:** Talika Line Solution
  I like this product. As well as 'filling' wrinkles it also 'fills' unsightly enlarged pores. It contains antioxidant vitamins A and

What's all the fuss about BB creams?

BB creams can actually be traced back to the 1950s when German Dr Christine Schrammek created a salve that was able to aid skin healing in post-peel and laser surgery patients while also camouflaging redness. Now, sixty years later, these creams are the hottest new trend and every skincare company seems to be developing one. The reason for their appeal is that BB creams (or Blemish Balms) claim to do everything, from moisturising and correcting skin tone to fighting spots and providing sun protection, meaning that, in theory, we don't need to spend time or money on lots of different skincare products. But do they actually do what they claim? Personally, I think you get better results by layering individual products, but they can be a good option if you're short on time, cash or shelf space. My favourite is Garnier's Miracle Skin Perfector Daily All-In-One BB Cream with SPF.

E, along with ceramides (naturally occurring fats that enable skin to retain water) and peptides.

- **High end:** Dermajuv Instant-Effect Lifting Serum
This is a pricey product, but it does have pretty impressive wrinkle-tightening results in just a few minutes. It's moisturising, too.

STEM CELLS IN SKIN CREAMS

Stem cells are the latest cutting edge ingredient in skincare. They can be taken from all living things – plants, animals and humans – and they have the remarkable ability to help repair tissue and rejuvenate skin. Stem cell creams mainly contain plant and fruit stem cells derived from apples, melons, roses or rice plants, in combination with other powerful anti-ageing ingredients such as peptides and pentapeptides. These creams are a great source of antioxidants and can help repair skin and restore its firmness by stimulating the production of new collagen and elastin. Try Harley Street Skin StemCellution Overnight Moisturiser, which contains a potent complex of fruit stem cells, antioxidants and peptides to stimulate cell growth and restore skin elasticity.

A WORD ABOUT SERUMS

Facial serums are fairly new to the skincare scene and, if you haven't got one, it's about time you began incorporating one into your routine. Serums are thinner and runnier than creams or lotions, allowing them to absorb more quickly, and they tend to have a higher concentration of powerful ingredients than other skin creams. Serums can vary in price from about £20 to more than £100, but they are well worth the investment as they include vitamins, antioxidants and/or acids to deliver results

such as fewer wrinkles, firmer skin, a brighter complexion a.
tion from environmental pollutants. My top choices are:

- Harley Street Skin StemCellution Anti-Ageing Serum, an amazing skin rejuvenator containing peptides and antioxidants that
  stimulate the production of collagen.
- Superdrug Swiss Apple Overnight Skin Renewal Serum, containing apple stem-cell extract to help reduce wrinkles.
- Boots No7 Protect & Perfect Beauty Serum to fight wrinkles.

FIRMING NECK CREAMS

Your neck is one of the first areas to show your age. This delicate skin tends
to wrinkle and head south very easily. Yet even though it's permanently on
show, it's often neglected when it comes to skincare and sunscreen – crazy!
Firming neck creams usually include antioxidant vitamins A, C and E,
AHAs and pigment inhibitors such as elderberry extract or lactic and tannic
acids to fade age spots, which can be a problem on necks. There are a few
ingredients like cecropia obtusa bark extract that help to discourage the
build-up of fatty tissue under the chin, AKA the dreaded turkey neck! They
may also contain peptides to boost cell regeneration.

My verdict: if you have a good anti-ageing day cream, I don't think it's
necessary to buy a separate neck product unless you want to. You may see
a little improvement with neck creams due to increased hydration and the
massage action when you rub them in, but I think you get the best effects
by using a good glycolic exfoliator along with your regular anti-ageing
moisturiser. The most important thing to do for the condition of your neck
skin is to extend your beauty regime from your face down to your bust.
Once turkey neck settles in, no cream will help shift it. It's time to bring
out the scarves and polo necks or consider a little surgical intervention.

My best buys

- **High street:** L'Oréal Advanced Revitalift Face & Neck Day Cream

  I really like this cream. It contains ingredients to smooth wrinkles, firm skin and provides long-lasting hydration.

- **High street:** Boots Time Delay Repair Face & Neck Moisturiser

  This great little cream protects against UV light, as well as having anti-ageing benefits. It's easy to pick up on most high streets and it smells nice, too!

- **High end:** Vexum.sl™ Double Chin Reducer

  The name promises a lot, but I like this product. It contains ingredients such as marine algae to tighten the skin and improve the appearance of sagging. It's worth a go, as long as your double chin is still at the developing stage.

BUST-FIRMING CREAMS

These creams obviously don't have the power to lift heavy breast tissue to give you those perky boobs you had in your 20s – they won't work miracles! However, they can help to improve things by firming tissue, adding moisture, and smoothing and tightening skin. I think massaging in these creams helps, but remember to massage upwards towards your neck.

They typically contain natural plant extracts to smooth and firm skin, as well as vitamins E and B to promote hydration and protect against free radicals.

My verdict: these creams can help boost the condition of your skin and are particularly useful for women after pregnancy or those who have lost weight. They can also improve the appearance of crêpey skin. However, massaging in any good moisturiser will help to improve your skin in this area.

My best buys

- **High street:** Palmer's Cocoa Butter Bust Firming Massage Cream With Vitamin E
  This smoothes on like a gel and is a great budget buy that's very popular with new mums.
- **Mid price:** Liz Earle Superskin Bust Treatment
  This light serum improves the skin's elasticity and tone and includes antioxidant vitamins.
- **High end:** Clarins Bust Beauty Extra-Lift Gel
  This is a refreshing gel formula that includes plant extracts to tighten and tone your skin.

TIP! Remember not to use bust-treatment creams while you're breast-feeding to avoid any ingredients being consumed by the baby.

FIRMING BODY MOISTURISERS

These hydrate the skin in the same way as a normal body cream to make skin look smoother and dewier, but they also contain anti-ageing ingredients such as collagen- and elastin-stimulating peptides, and antioxidants including vitamin E.

My verdict: any creams with added anti-ageing ingredients are probably more effective than your bog-standard moisturiser, but don't expect dramatic results. A good choice for new mums who want to improve skin tone after the birth.

My best buys

- **High street:** Vaseline Firming & Nourishing Lotion

An apple a day to keep wrinkles at bay

Apples are the next big anti-ageing ingredient. Not just any old apple, mind, but a rare Swiss apple from the Uttwiler Spatlauber. High-end creams that contain it already have an A-list following and even First Lady, Michelle Obama, is said to use an expensive skin serum with an extract from the stem cells of this apple.

Apparently the variety stays fresh for up to four months after being harvested, long after other varieties have shrivelled up. It's believed stem cells from the fruit can stimulate human skin stem cells, thereby protecting skin cell regeneration and delaying the onset of wrinkles.

Apples are also rich in antioxidant flavonoids, which can protect against environmental damage to the skin, as well as phenols, which provide UVB protection, making skin more resistant to sun damage. Braeburn, Fuji and Red Delicious are all rich in phenols.

However, with Uttwiler Spatlauber apple creams costing around £200 (this discovery is yet to find its way into high street products), for the moment I'd rather eat apples than put them on my face!

This good-value product is super-moisturising and has peptides to restore elasticity. A great bargain buy.

- **Mid price:** Clarins Body Firming Cream
This cream uses silicon and botanicals such as gingko biloba to firm and nourish. With regular use, skin becomes smoother and more toned over time.

- **High end:** Gatineau Melatogenine Body Intensive Firming Cream
  This contains antioxidants as well as a unique trademarked molecule called Melatogenine™ to firm skin.

CELLULITE CREAMS

If a tube of cream could get rid of cellulite, there would be millions of very happy women out there. Unfortunately, nothing's going to shift those dreaded lumps and bumps permanently apart from a healthy diet, tons of water and exercise – and even then you might have problem areas. What some creams can do, however, is smooth the surface of your skin temporarily, aided by the massage action of applying them. They typically contain antioxidants and caffeine to stimulate circulation.

My verdict: there's no harm in using these creams to keep your thighs smooth and hydrated, but any cellulite-busting effects are temporary. Bear this in mind before splashing out on a fancy product. Cellulite is stubborn stuff and the only quick way to get rid of it is to try liposuction or less invasive techniques such as CelluTite, Cellulaze or BodyTite™. But even though these will remove fat, you can still be left with the 'orange peel' effect – even slim women get cellulite! For more on this, see page 233.

The other option, of course, is to hold in the bulges with thigh-firming pants (see page 236).

My best buys
- **Mid price:** Revitol Cellulite Solution
  This contains caffeine and vitamin-A derivative retinol, so it works on circulation as well as helping to improve the texture of your skin and stimulate collagen. It also includes algae for skin firming.
- **Mid price:** Liz Earle Energising Hip And Thigh Gel
  This uses natural active ingredients such as butcher's broom,

horse chestnut, rosemary and geranium to reduce puffiness and boost circulation. It feels nice and cool when it goes on and skin feels tighter as it dries.

- **High end:** Medik8 Lipomelt Forte

This one's my favourite. It uses caffeine to boost circulation and coenzyme A, which is thought to help break down fat. It's absorbed really quickly, but you should wait until it's dry before applying your regular body cream.

MIRACLE GADGETS

The beauty business is constantly trying to come up with clever new products to keep us looking younger and there's a growing trend for anti-ageing devices to use at home that mimic salon or clinic technology. Most of them are pretty pricey (anything from £50 to a few hundred pounds), but can they actually make a difference? I tried a few to see what they're all about.

Dermaroller Home Meso-rejuvenation device

This roller, covered in tiny needles, is based on the micro-needling treatment we use in clinics (see page 177). The principle is the same – you roll the device over your skin so the needles penetrate, inducing enough damage so the skin's own repair mechanism kicks into gear, increasing collagen and elastin. It also allows anti-ageing skincare products to penetrate deeper.

You have to roll the Dermaroller vertically and horizontally over your entire face, which is quite hard to do yourself – and it hurts! I'm not sure you'd get deep enough penetration from the needles for it to be effective. I think it's fantastic as a clinic treatment but, if you want to try it at home, have a professional treatment first and ask your practitioner to show you how to do it properly.

It's very important to clean the Dermaroller properly and it's not suitable if you have active acne, infected skin, eczema, psoriasis, rosacea, open wounds or sores, raised moles or warts.

The Tua Tre'nd

This hand-held gadget uses electrical impulses to tone face and neck muscles and to stimulate the skin. It takes around half an hour to do your whole face or you can target specific areas.

I've tried many of these 'facial toning' devices over the years – from Cleo, one of the first available brands, through to ilift (see opposite). My opinion is that a device like Tua Tre'nd would need to be used every day, even up to twice a day, to see results and, if you stop using it for a few days, the benefits will be lost. This is one for women with staying power!

Rejuve magnetic mask

I like the idea of this mask with magnets which increase circulation to regenerate the skin. I think it could work if used regularly, but – and this is a very big but – who on earth has three or four hours a day to wear one of these masks, only to wait three or four weeks for results? You can wear it through the night (but forget your sex life). This one's a non-starter for me.

Facial-Flex

This facial exercise device, available from Rosemary Conley's website (see page 278), is designed to tone up areas prone to sagging, such as the jawline. It's probably my favourite at-home anti-ageing gadget because it can get results and it doesn't cost the earth.

I'm all for facial exercises. They're not time-consuming and you can do them almost anywhere. You simply fit this gadget – which is held together with elastic bands in the middle – into the corners of your mouth and do two minutes of repetitive exercises. As well as tightening muscles it'll do a bit for the skin too as it's improving circulation.

BEST FOR VALUE: Slendertone Face

This works by stimulating the muscles that support the fine facial skin, firming them so the face looks plumper and more youthful. As our muscles become less firm with age the skin has less structure and starts to hang. It's exercise again, but a gadget does it for you. I think this is a good machine that works well with regular use.

ilift anti-ageing, skin rejuvenation device

I really like this little hand-held device to improve skin firmness and tone. Infrared light stimulates collagen and improves circulation, while the massage action boosts skin elasticity and firms the supporting muscles. You need to use it for about 20 minutes a day. I've tried this gadget and really like it. It can give a gentle lift with regular use. You'll get better results if you can use it twice a day.

MY TOP BUY: Therapulse

This is a seriously good machine – and a serious investment. The other devices I've mentioned will set you back a couple of hundred pounds for the most expensive ones, but this is a whopping £3,500. It was developed in the medical arena and has the ability to change skin tone and texture. It can reduce wrinkles around the eyes, and tone muscles. It also stimulates the body's own natural production of VEGF – a natural growth factor that helps repair and regenerate the skin. You can even use it on your legs to improve firmness and reduce cellulite.

The treatment works by delivering low-voltage impulses through the skin via electrodes positioned on the area to be treated. It doesn't hurt and you should start seeing results after a couple of sessions when your skin starts to look brighter and tighter.

six

Get a More Youthful Face

When it comes to ageing we tend to think of the face first and all those nasty little surprises that creep up on us when we're not paying attention – eye bags, crow's feet, frown lines, jowls, wrinkles, to name just a few! Not much to look forward to – right, ladies? That's why it always amazes me how many women are willing to spend a fortune on designer hand-bags and take hours agonising over their outfits, but pay so little attention to the skin on their faces. That's definitely the wrong way round.

Unlike the latest 'it' bag, your face needs to last you a lifetime. You have to invest in it – and I'm not talking about spending money on cosmetic treatments once the wrinkles have settled in. You need to treat your face with tender loving care, develop a good skincare regime, and protect it from the ageing effects of the sun to stay looking fabulous as the years go by.

After all, your face is your best asset. We all know how positively we respond to someone who has a beautiful warm smile, glowing healthy skin and gorgeous sparkly eyes. And, more importantly, if you feel good about how you look, it gives you amazing confidence to tackle the world.

Unfortunately, none of us can escape those signs of ageing – they get round to us all eventually. When I reached my early 40s, I started thinking seriously about having anti-ageing treatments. I still felt 25, of course, but one day I was confronted by the cold, hard truth in the form of a new passport photo. When I looked at it I thought, 'God, there she is – my mum!' The eye bags were starting to develop and my neck was a little heavier. People had begun telling me how much I looked like my mother, too. Now, don't misunderstand me – my mum is gorgeous. But she was 70 at the time and I wasn't ready to fast-forward three decades.

Luckily, there is a lot we can do to stay looking younger for longer. In this chapter I'm going to arm you with all the options for tackling problems in each area of the face, from DIY fixes and non-invasive clinic treatments right through to last-resort surgical methods.

So read on for all my best tips, tricks and insider advice to hold back the years and keep your face looking radiant and fresh for as long as possible.

The problem: eye wrinkles

You can tell a lot about a person by looking at their eyes. They really are the windows to the soul. Unfortunately, the skin around your eyes is usually the first to show signs of ageing because it's thinner and has fewer oil glands, making it drier and more vulnerable to wrinkles. I always think a few little lines around the eyes add character, but too many will make you look haggard. I liked my face in my 30s when I had a few laughter lines, but when I hit 40 I wanted to get rid of the crow's feet. Here's how to tackle them.

DIY FIXES

Sunglasses – don't leave home without them!

Have you noticed that celebrities always wear huge oversized sunglasses? It's not just because they're fashionable and look great in paparazzi pictures; they also protect your eyes from those ageing UVA rays, which break down collagen and cause wrinkles. They'll stop you screwing up your eyes in bright sunlight, which causes crinkles around your eyes and nose. Look out for styles that block both UVA and UVB rays – and remember, if you want to look ultra-glam, the bigger the better!

Try a good eye cream

There are some decent eye creams containing wrinkle-relaxing peptides that smooth lines if you use them regularly. I like Marks & Spencer Formula Age Repair Ceramide Eye Cream. You could try a 'filler' cream such as Olay's Regenerist 30 Second Wrinkle Filler, which temporarily 'fills' lines. I also like Natural Skin Solutions Instant Eye Lift, which eases wrinkles, tightens skin and includes UVB protection. But my all-time favourite all-round eye cream is Jan Marini C-ESTA® Eye Repair Concentrate. It's a fantastic product that helps to firm and tighten the whole eye area and reduce fine lines. For more on eye creams, see page 116.

> **TIP!** It's hard to find eye creams with sun protection to wear during the day, so I developed one called Eye Refining Serum with an SPF 8. The alternative is to use mineral make-up, such as BPC's Mineral Pressed Foundation, which includes a natural sunscreen.

Try glycolic acid

There are very few eye creams containing glycolic acid, which is an effective ingredient for removing the layers of dead skin that make wrinkles look deeper. My favourite is Jan Marini Bioglycolic® Eye Cream.

Glycolic acid is quite a powerful ingredient, though, so use eye creams that contain it sparingly – I'd suggest every second day. And always follow with a sunscreen to protect the newer skin from damaging rays.

> **TIP!** To tighten the skin underneath your eyes, I've found this home-made eye mask works wonders before a night out. Crack an egg and divide the egg white from the yolk. Using cotton wool, apply the egg white to your wrinkles and leave for 15 minutes. You'll feel your skin tightening as the egg white hardens. Using lukewarm water, gently wash the area, pat dry and you're ready for your close-up! The effect will last for an evening.

AT THE CLINIC

Botox

This is very effective at banishing crow's feet when it's injected into the muscles around the outer corners of your eye. My advice would be to use small amounts for a more natural effect. If it's your first treatment, follow the 'less is more' rule – you can always have a top-up.

Ouch factor: not painful, but you might experience a slight pinching or burning during the injections.

How long will it last? Three to six months.

Pellevé

Pellevé is the latest groundbreaking anti-ageing treatment and is a great way to diminish fine lines around the eyes. It uses radiofrequency waves

DID YOU KNOW? Botox is a brand name for a botulinum toxin. When small amounts are injected under the surface of the skin, the muscles relax, causing skin to lie smoothly and wrinkles to disappear. It's one of the most popular treatments at our clinic – and in the UK. These days there are lots of different brands on the market. My preferred toxin is called Azzalure®. It has a quick effect and used in tiny amounts can have a stunning effect on the face. For more on Botox, see pages 149–50.

to stimulate collagen production. One treatment will give instant results but two to three will give lasting effects.

Ouch factor: not painful and no downtime is needed following treatment.

How long will it last? A course of three treatments will last up to a year.

Fillers

These can be used to get rid of crow's feet. A light filler such as Restylane® Touch, Restylane® Vital or Teosyal® can be injected underneath the lines to fill them out. Both of these fillers contain hyaluronic acid, which occurs naturally in the body, so you're less likely to have a reaction to them.

Ouch factor: can be a little painful, but your doctor will use a topical anaesthetic 40 minutes before the treatment. Restylane® has a local anaesthetic in it, so once the treatment starts you won't feel it.

How long will it last? Six to twelve months

Microdermabrasion

This deep exfoliating facial gets rid of dead skin cells and plumps up skin by stimulating collagen. It's not a favourite of mine, though. The only one I like using on our clients is Naturepeel, as it uses salt to sandblast the skin instead of aluminium crystals, which I think are too abrasive and can be a nightmare to remove from eyes, nose and hair. Salt just melts away and is actually healing to the skin. The upside is that microdermabrasion improves the condition of your whole complexion instead of just target-ing specific wrinkles around your eyes, the way Botox and fillers do.

I would only use this treatment around the corners of the eyes.

Your face is cleansed first, eye shields are popped on, then a nozzle shoots fine crystals of aluminium or salt against the skin to loosen dead skin cells. Your face is cleansed and moisturised afterwards.

Ouch factor: gentle tingling.

How long will it last? You'll need a course of six, then top-up treat-ments every few months for lasting benefits. A one-off treatment is a good skin boost for a special event.

Intense pulsed light (IPL)

This helps ease fine lines and get rid of sun damage around the eyes. The light from a computer-controlled lamp penetrates the skin, heating up cells and stimulating collagen. It works best on fair skins, though, and you shouldn't have it if you've recently had a suntan, as you could end up with uneven skin tone. This treatment can have good results, but make sure you go to a reputable clinic as I've seen people who've been burnt with IPL.

Ouch factor: it can hurt!

How long will it last? Up to three months.

Gentle peels

A light chemical peel can help smooth lines and hydrate the delicate eye area. Glycolic acid peels are my favourite. I'd go for one containing 40% or less of glycolic acid. In my experience it's better to have a weaker peel over six to eight weeks than a one-off treatment that's more intense. My favourite is Jan Marini 40%, which helps with sun damage, too; it's a good option if you want to boost your whole complexion, as well as target wrinkles around your eyes.

For more on chemical peels, see pages 167–8.

Ouch factor: gentle tingling

How long will it last? I'd advise a peel once a week for six weeks to get the best results, then a monthly top-up a couple of months after you've finished the course. Or you could use an at-home glycolic peel to maintain the effects. I like NeoStrata Citriate Home Skin Peel. The effects from a one-off treatment will last for about four days.

> **TIP!** Always prepare your skin for a peel by using beauty products containing glycolic acid for two weeks beforehand. NeoStrata is a good range – try the Foaming Glycolic Wash followed either by the Ultra Daytime Smoothing Cream SPF 15 or Ultra Moisturizing Face Cream at night. This is a gentle introduction for first timers to treatments that change the way your skin feels, behaves and looks.

Laser resurfacing

This is excellent for tightening the skin around the eyes, but it's not for the faint-hearted. It's a serious treatment in which a laser pierces thousands of tiny holes in the skin. This makes your skin produce collagen to heal the piercings, so it becomes thicker. You may need three treatments a month apart, but it can turn back the clock ten years on your skin.

Ouch factor: it can really hurt, even with an anaesthetic, but the results are great.

How long will it last? Up to ten years.

For advice on choosing a clinic for non-surgical treatments, including injectables, lasers and peels, see pages 178–82.

The problems: puffy eyes and bags

Nothing is more ageing than looking as though you're carrying two bags of shopping underneath your peepers! Sometimes surgery is the only option when it comes to eye bags that develop with age. Over the years, the fat under your eye moves down and forms a ridge, which is incredibly ageing. If your parents have them, the chances are that's what's in store for you. I always advise my patients to have this done sooner rather than later for the best results. See page 182 for Nip Tuck advice. But first of all, try my road-tested suggestions below if puffy, baggy eyes are your beauty *bête noire*.

DIY FIXES

Try massage

With your ring finger, gently massage in a circular motion from the inner corner of your eye towards your temple. Do this every morning to help disperse fluid and reduce puffiness.

Get cold comfort

Wrap an ice cube in a cotton handkerchief or a piece of muslin and gently press it underneath your eyes to reduce puffiness. Or try that supermodel trick of placing chilled teaspoons over your eyes. Gel-filled masks, which you can pick up at most pharmacies, are useful to keep in the fridge for eye-bag emergencies!

Brew a soothing cuppa

Dip cotton pads in brewed white or green tea. Gently squeeze out the excess fluid, then place the pads in a covered container in the fridge for between 30 and 60 minutes. Place the pads on your eyes, then lie back and relax for 20 minutes.

Feed the problem

Thin slices of cold cucumber or raw potato placed over closed eyes work well at reducing puffiness from too much partying! If you have the time, make a home-made mask by blending the cucumber or potato in a food processor until it forms a thick paste, then put it in the fridge to chill. Apply the mask carefully around your eyes, taking care not to get any of it in the eyes.

Buy more pillows!

When you lie down to sleep, the water in your body levels out and settles underneath your eyes, causing puffiness. Sleep on your back and raise your head by propping it on a couple of pillows, which will help the fluid to drain away. When patients have eye surgery at our clinic, we recommend they sleep for a week propped up on pillows.

Bounce bags away

Buy a mini-trampoline – I'm not joking! Bouncing up and down will help drain the fluid that causes puffiness. Dancing and jogging work, too.

Watch your diet

Salt causes water retention, so to help combat fluid gathering under your eyes, cut down on it. Processed foods and ready-meals contain lots of hidden salt, so try to eliminate these from your diet.

Try a treatment mask

Masks are much more effective than eye creams or gels at getting rid of puffy eyes and are a good rescue remedy after a heavy night. One of my favourites is Talika Eye Decompress, which soothes, refreshes and helps bring down puffiness.

> **TIP!** If you can't afford to buy a separate eye cream, my view is that you don't have to. A good anti-ageing day cream, as long as it's a light serum, will do just as well.

For more on eye creams, see page 116.

AT THE CLINIC

Radiofrequency modelling

A treatment called Radiage is great for tightening baggy eyes. A cool gel is applied first, then a Radiage 'wand' is used to heat up the site. It uses radio frequency energy to heat up the soft tissue beneath the skin, causing collagen to contract and tighten.

Ouch factor: it's not painful, but it might take a couple of weeks for the redness to disappear.

How long will it last? It can last up to four years depending on your age and skin type, with six-monthly top-ups. I'd recommend a course of three initial treatments, two weeks apart.

The problem: dark circles

The panda look isn't flattering on anyone, but fortunately there are plenty of fixes you can try.

DIY FIXES

Find a good concealer

Choose a formula that's designed to be used under the eyes (these usually come in a pump dispenser with a brush attached or with a wand applicator). Avoid thick, drier formulas that come in pots, as these are more suited to covering blemishes. And choose one that's a shade lighter than your natural skin colour.

Once you've applied it to the dark areas, dab it gently with your finger-tip to blend it in. Don't wipe it on as you'll actually just be wiping it off!

Try YSL Touche Éclat – this light-reflective under-eye miracle worker makes it into the best beauty products lists in magazines year after year.

A personal favourite of mine is Bourjois Light Reflecting Concealer, which is a fraction of the cost of some other brands, but works just as well.

Two more clever little products are Benefit Ooh La Lift, a brightening pink balm for under the eyes and Benefit Powderflage, a super-fine powder with light-reflecting particles that you can use alone or over your regular concealer for greater coverage.

I also like BPC Camofleur, a really light cream-to-powder concealer with light-reflecting minerals and a natural SPF 20.

Get your beauty sleep!

Dark circles are usually the result of too many late nights. If you've been burning the candle at both ends, examine your lifestyle and decide what you can change to help you get more sleep. If you can manage to get to bed at 10pm at least twice a week, that's a good start. If insomnia is the problem, you could benefit from de-stressing some parts of your life and learning a few relaxation techniques. For more on this, see pages 69–79.

Come out of the shadows

Try NeoStrata Bionic Eye Cream. This targets under-eye shadows, evening out skin tone and brightening and smoothing the whole area. It feels nice around your eyes, too. Worth a go if you feel like splashing out on a special eye product.

AT THE CLINIC

Radiage

As well as tightening baggy eyes, this radiofrequency treatment can also help with dark circles. Because the skin is so thin underneath your eye, it's often a vein that you see rather than a dark circle. Radiage helps by stimulating collagen and thickening the skin so you can't see the vein.

Ouch factor: not painful

How long will it last? Several years, with regular top-ups.

> **TIP!** I see a lot of Asian women at the clinic who suffer with terrible dark circles, which affect their self-confidence. Radiage can help, but I've had great success with a skin-brightening peptide cream called ZO Brightenex™, which is also great at treating hyperpigmentation (darker patches of skin caused by sun damage or acne). See page 163 for more on this.

The problem: tear troughs

These nasty hollows run from the inner corners of your eyes to the top of the cheeks, almost cutting the cheek pads in two. Even the name is depressing! They're usually genetic and largely down to ageing and losing fat from the upper cheeks (just under your lower eyelids), as well as sagging of the cheek's upper muscles. The result? You look tired, old and miserable!

Other than being very clever with light-reflecting make-up and under-eye concealer, there aren't any DIY tricks to combat tear troughs. You can help prevent them by keeping your weight steady. Losing too much fat from your face will only make them stand out more.

AT THE CLINIC

Restylane®

Restylane® is seen by many practitioners as the gold standard in aesthetic injectables and it works well for tear troughs. It is made from hyaluronic acid, which occurs naturally in the skin, and is injected with an incredibly fine needle to counteract the loss of fat in the tear troughs. It works well in this delicate area because it is light and malleable so you don't get lumps. It also contains lidocaine anaesthetic, which reduces any pain caused by treatment.

Ouch factor: minimal.

How long will it last? One treatment will last up to six months.

The problem: droopy brow

A sagging forehead can affect the expression in your eyes and make you look depressed and/or worried. Here are some methods that can give you a lift.

DIY FIXES

Get a clever up-do

For an instant brow lift that costs nothing and doesn't hurt a bit, pull your hair back tightly into a high ponytail. It really does help to get rid of that hang-dog expression!

Get your eyebrows shaped

This is a simple thing to do, but it can 'lift' your whole face, opening up your eyes and making you look years younger. Have your eyebrows waxed professionally to get the right shape, then it's easier to pluck them yourself at home. For the best results, invest in a good, sharp pair of tweezers. Make-up artists and models swear by Tweezerman and I like them, too. Or try Eylure Brow Beauty Kit, which includes stencils to get the perfect shape, tweezers and defining pencils for blondes and brunettes.

Curl your lashes

This will give your eyes a brighter, more wide-awake look. Don't bother with pricey heated eyelash curlers, though – if you give your regular eyelash curlers a blast with the hairdryer, they'll do the job just as well. Make sure they're not too hot before using them!

Lighten up!

Clever use of concealer on your lids and brow bone can brighten up your eyes and make the whole area appear instantly younger. Choose a shade lighter than your skin then, using a small brush, apply the concealer under your eyebrows and blend in. Next, apply it to your lids and blend in gently. Benefit has a great 'brow-lifting' pencil called High Brow in a soft pink shade, which you apply under your brows following the arch. Perfect when you need to look as though you've had a full eight hours' sleep when you've only had four!

For a more glamorous evening look, try applying a little face highlighter that has a slight shimmer underneath your brows.

AT THE CLINIC

Botox brow lift

Small amounts of Botox are injected into the brows so the 'down pulling' muscles are relaxed and the 'up pulling' muscles can work more efficiently, raising your brows. In some cases it can raise the upper lids slightly, too.

Ouch factor: not painful.
How long will it last? Three to six months.

Laser resurfacing

My preferred laser for this would be Fraxel Repair, which uses carbon dioxide laser beams to penetrate the skin, creating thousands of microscopic wounds to stimulate collagen and tighten the skin. It all sounds a bit space age, I admit, but this treatment can shrink back your skin, lifting your brow and getting rid of that careworn look. It takes about a week for your skin to recover and it'll be very red and flaky, but if you can take a week off to have this treatment, the results are excellent.
Ouch factor: there's no getting round it, this can be painful!
How long will it last? Two to five years.

A *word about ears!*

I bet you didn't know this: as you age your ears start to droop and you can get flat saggy lobes. The problem is often worse if you've worn chandelier earrings your whole life. It's not a good look when you want to put your hair up or tuck it behind your ears. The good news is, you can have a filler injected to plump them up again. It can be a painful place to inject so a topical anaesthetic is applied to the lobe for about 40 minutes beforehand, then a small amount of filler is injected to replace volume. Earrings can be worn the very next day and it lasts about a year.

The problems: forehead wrinkles and frown furrow

Forehead wrinkles are very ageing. They can make you look as though you have the cares of the world on your shoulders. And those 'number 11' lines between your eyes, which are brought on by repetitive frowning, make you appear mean and angry. It's the area many women are most bothered about – certainly among the women who come to our clinic. And it seems we'll resort to all kinds of DIY methods to make them less obvious. I remember my mum telling me that years ago women used to put Sellotape across their foreheads before getting into bed in the hope it would smooth their wrinkles overnight. Not sure that approach would do much for your love life, though! Luckily, these days we have a few more options. Here are some ideas for a younger look.

DIY FIXES

Paper over the cracks

Try Frownies. These brown paper facial patches are legendary in the beauty business. They aim to retrain your muscles so you stop frowning (using the same principle as the Sellotape trick). You simply dampen them with water and apply to wrinkles. For the best results, wear them for 30 days at first, preferably overnight. Worth a try if you have the patience to persevere – and a lot cheaper than Botox! But maybe save them till you're on you're own; like Sellotape, they're not sexy!

Stop squinting

If you squint a lot to read or watch the telly, pay a visit to your optician. You could need glasses, or a change of prescription if you already have some. Repetitive squinting will only deepen those forehead furrows.

Grow a fringe!

It's cheap and could be just what you need to revamp your look. Make sure your hairdresser cuts into the ends of your fringe to soften it. A blunt line is too harsh if you're older.

Fill in the gaps

Benefit has a clever product called Dr Feelgood, which is a colourless balm you smooth on with a sponge to fill in fine lines and get rid of shine. You can wear it over make-up or alone. It's a good temporary fix for smoothing a furrowed forehead after a late night.

And relax...

As well as a good anti-ageing moisturiser to help plump up lines and keep skin hydrated, you could try a serum with a muscle-relaxing peptide such as Argireline (acetyl hexapeptide-3), which is often touted as an alternative to Botox, although it's nowhere near as effective. You need to use such a cream for 30 days to see the best results and you have to apply it religiously twice a day. Within 24 hours of not using it those lines will quickly reappear. It's worth a try if you're bothered by wrinkles but don't feel ready to go down the Botox route. (For more on Botox, see below.)

AT THE CLINIC

Botox

This is without doubt the best clinic treatment for forehead wrinkles, as fillers can look raised and obvious. One treatment is usually given over two sessions. During the second appointment two to four weeks after the first, the doctor will assess your skin to see if you need a top-up.

Contrary to what a lot of people think, you can have Botox (and other toxins such as Azzalure®) and still retain movement in your forehead. The

My take on Botox

Although it's become a hugely popular treatment, the muscle-relaxing effect of Botox isn't for everyone. Personally, I hate the feeling of not being able to move my face, so I have only tiny amounts for a slightly relaxed look that's very natural and still lets me have expressions. If I'm surprised people know and if I'm cross people know! That's the way it should be. The key to good, natural results with Botox is to use it sparingly – and this is the approach any good cosmetic doctor will take.

As I've mentioned before, Botox is actually a trade name; there are other botulinum toxins available, such as Azzalure® and Dysport®.

I don't have any safety concerns when it comes to botulinum toxins, as they've been used for more than 30 years in the medical arena to treat everything from migraine to muscle spasms. The only danger comes when Botox is obtained from unreliable sources, such as over the Internet, or administered in huge doses. This would be the case with any drug. If you go to a reputable clinic, you have no reason to worry (see pages 178–82 for advice on choosing a clinic).

For me, the biggest downside is that when Botox wears off – which it does after between three and six months – you'll return to how you looked before and having regular top-ups can get expensive.

However, if you have tiny amounts of Botox injected every few months for up to seven years, it'll re-educate your muscles so they get out of the habit of moving the way they did and eventually you won't need it any more. Used this way, it can arrest signs of ageing such as brow droop and deep forehead furrows.

key is to have small amounts, just enough to soften lines – we call it Micro-tox at our clinic. With tiny amounts you don't risk getting those permanently surprised Mr Spock eyebrows or a big shiny, frozen forehead. **Ouch factor:** not painful.

How long will it last? You'll see the effects for between three and six months.

Problem: loss of lip volume

Full lips have always been associated with youth and beauty. What woman wouldn't want a super-sexy pout like Angelina Jolie's? Sadly, as we get older our lips lose their pillowy plumpness and the tissue around them loses volume, too. The bone above the teeth also starts to shrink back so the lips have less support and begin to curl inwards.

The good news is, there's loads you can do these days to restore some plumpness, whether it's tricking the eye with make-up, applying some clever creams or paying a visit to a clinic to take advantage of the latest non-surgical techniques.

Years ago, cosmetic doctors used to plump up lips by making two tiny incisions on either side of the mouth and threading a cord through the outline of your lips. Often the incisions would get infected or take ages to heal. Thankfully, techniques have come a long way since then with temporary injectable fillers that can give a subtle plumping effect that looks very natural. Here are my tips on reclaiming your pout.

DIY FIXES

Get an instant pout

If you're looking for a temporary fix, lip-plumping primers and glosses can give the appearance of fuller lips. Primers come in neutral shades and fill in fine lines, which helps to prevent lipstick bleed and makes your lip colour last longer, too. Try Benefit Lip Plump.

Plumping glosses are also popular. Go for a light formula that's moisturising and non-sticky. Try Laura Mercier Lip Plumper in a shade called Lychee, a neutral (almost clear) colour that you can wear alone or over lipstick. It suits all skin tones.

For ongoing benefits, use a lip-plumping cream as part of your regular beauty regime and smooth it over lips and around the contours of your mouth. Try Elizabeth Arden Ceramide Plump Perfect Lip Moisture Cream SPF 30. It contains the peptide Argireline to soften lines, a lip-plumping ingredient and a sunscreen (SPF always gets a gold star from me).

Add moisture

Dry, cracked lips look thin (and old) so always keep a good lip balm handy to lock in moisture. This will prevent them getting dried out by the sun in summer and by cold air, harsh winds and central heating in winter.

I love a product called Lip Spa by BPC Mineral Make-up, which includes two products, Lip Pumice and Lip Treat. The pumice is an exfoliator, which you massage into your lips with a damp finger, and the treat is a stick of pure vitamin E, which is moisturing and anti-ageing. It's one of my beauty bag essentials.

> **TIP!** For a DIY lip exfoliator, add a little olive oil to some sugar and rub it gently over your lips to get rid of flakiness and leave them super-smooth.

Get clever with make-up

Cleverly applied lipstick and liner combined with a few little highlighting tricks can deceive the eye, making it look as though you have fuller lips – and it's pretty easy to do.

For an evening look, use a primer in a nude shade to 'fill' lines and help prevent the colour bleeding, then apply your lipstick with a brush. It's best to go for a moisturising lipstick with a slight sheen or gloss rather than one with a matte finish, which I think looks too harsh. If you're older, steer clear of darker shades as these are incredibly ageing. Pinks and neutral tones work best (for more make-up tricks, see pages 88–96).

Next, take a lip liner pencil that's as close to your lipstick shade as possible and lightly push it around your lipline in short strokes – never 'draw' it on. Finally, apply a little shimmering gloss to the middle of both lips and you're ready to hit the town.

For a more natural pout that looks good for daytime, go for a lip-plumping gloss in a natural shade. First, apply a nude lip liner in light feathery strokes, then smooth on your gloss with a brush or wand applicator. To make your upper lip appear fuller, use a white pencil or a nude shade with a shimmer effect just above the V of your Cupid's bow. To make your bottom lip seem plumper, add a little shimmering gloss or face highlighting powder to the centre of it.

AT THE CLINIC

Fillers

Plumping up lips with fillers is a popular treatment now, probably because so many celebs have it done and the results look good on most. Treatments have come on leaps and bounds in recent years and a good doctor can achieve a very natural effect. Fillers can be injected into the lip body to make your mouth a little fuller and around the edge of the lips (what's known as the vermilion border), which smoothes out small lines instantly.

Most practitioners in the UK use hyaluronic acid-based products and my filler of choice is Restylane®. I like it because it's been tried and tested over several years and has a local anaesthetic in it so the ouch factor is reduced.

After a treatment most people have some redness, swelling and tenderness in the area or even a small bruise, which can last up to a week. My advice is always to have these treatments when you're not doing anything desperately important, just in case things take a few days to settle down. If you need to cover redness or bruising, use mineral make-up, which won't cause infection.

Ouch factor: a little uncomfortable.

How long will it last? This depends on how efficiently your body disposes of the filler. Most hyaluronic acid fillers will last between six and nine months but at the clinic we've noticed it can last a year or even 18 months in some people.

How can I avoid a 'trout pout'?

Q: I'm 40 and look pretty good for my age, except my lips seem to have got thinner over the years. I'd like to have a filler to plump them up but I'm worried about getting a trout pout after seeing a couple of celebrities with over-inflated lips. What's your advice?

A: Ask your doctor to put in the minimum amount of filler to start with so you can see how you like it. You can always get more next time. If you have loads to begin with and don't like the effect, that's where you'll run into trouble because it'll take several months for the filler to be absorbed and disappear.

A good doctor or dermatologist will be interested in having a long-term relationship with you and caring for your skin as it changes over the years, and they'll want to achieve a subtle, natural look.

My philosophy has always been to build up gradually so patients don't leave the clinic looking completely different – that would be a huge shock for them and for everyone who knows them. It's a bit like having a drastic haircut. If you go from having shoulder-length hair to a super-short crop, it can be a shock to see yourself looking so different. If you'd built up to that crop gradually, it wouldn't seem like such a huge change. Likewise, if you have a lip-plumping treatment that leaves you looking completely different, it's going to take some getting used to. That's why I recommend taking it slowly.

I prefer a hyarulonic acid-based filler. I've been using this to add a little subtle volume to my lips for around 15 years and have always been very happy with the results.

A word of warning: never, ever have a permanent synthetic filler such as silicone put into your lips because once it's in place, it's impossible to remove. So if you had an allergic reaction, causing your lips to swell up, or if you didn't like the effect, you would be stuck with it. You might be tempted by a permanent solution given the cost of having your lips done every few months, but remember that it could cost you your looks if you end up with a permanent trout pout.

You should also think about what you'll look like 20 years from now. That permanent lip job may look OK at the moment, but will probably look pretty odd when you're a pensioner.

The only permanent solution I'd ever consider is injections of your own fat and stem cells (taken from your thighs) to plump up lips. This is a fairly new treatment, so it's still expensive, but the results are ever-lasting and your lips will age naturally with you.

TIP! If you want to see what you'd look like with a fuller pout, have a Cinderella Lips treatment in which saline is injected into your lipline. It takes 20 minutes and you'll be given a dental block to anaesthetise your mouth. The effects last just 48 hours – good news if you don't like it! It's a great quick-fix treatment for a special event. I know loads of celebrities who have this before hitting the red carpet.

The problem: pucker lines

As we age, some of us start to develop those nasty lines that run vertically across the top lip, known in the trade as pucker lines. You can see these lines if you look in the mirror and pucker up as if you're about to kiss someone. As we get older, these become permanent and are incredibly ageing, particularly when your lipstick starts to bleed into them. But never fear – there are solutions.

DIY FIXES

Stop smoking (or don't start)
The people with the worst pucker lines are smokers who've spent years sucking on cigarettes. It's one of the hardest areas to treat once the damage has been done, so be warned.

Avoid drinking from a straw!
Hopefully you've grown out of this by now but, if you're a cocktail fan, get rid of the straw when your mojito arrives!

Don't forget TLC

I'm amazed how many women neglect the upper lip area. It often gets missed out when it comes to cleansing and moisturising. I know this because when women come to me for a consultation, I analyse their skin using a computer and there are often a lot of bacteria across this area. There's not much flesh there and it ages faster than some other areas, so you have to pay it attention. Using a good cream with peptides (to support collagen and elastin and plump out fine lines), and AHAs (to get rid of dead skin cells) will help this area look smoother and more youthful.

Try a ridge filler cream

Creams and serums that target specific wrinkles can provide a quick fix as well as reducing the appearance of lines if used regularly, although they won't shift trenches! My favourite is Jan Marini C-ESTA® Lips, which works well on fine lines above your top lip and is also useful for the deeper furrows that run from the nose to your top lip. I've used it on several occasions as an emergency fix to plump up this area before an evening out.

AT THE CLINIC

Laser resurfacing

This is the best treatment for these hard-to-shift lines, particularly if they're deeply ingrained from years of smoking or sun damage. As well as stimulating collagen production to thicken the skin and dramatically reduce lines, it tightens the area, too.

Ouch factor: be prepared – it can hurt! You'll need downtime of up to seven days until the redness disappears, so it's best to clear your diary.

How long will it last? Between two and five years.

Botox and fillers

Toxins such as Botox or Azzalure® can work for this area if they're used in teeny-tiny amounts, but choose a very experienced practitioner to do it or you could end up with a droopy mouth. When filler is used here it tends to be visible, and can end up looking worse than the lines you were trying to get rid of. However, there is a filler called Restylane® Vital, a very fine form of hyaluronic acid, which can be criss-crossed across the top lip. You may need three treatments, two weeks apart, and it would need to be redone every year.

The problem: nose-to-mouth lines

As we age, nose-to-mouth lines become deeper. These are the lines that run from each side of your nose out towards the corners of your mouth. I like to call them 'smile lines' as it sounds nicer! They can be more obvious if you've lost or put on weight and can look deeper on one side. Here's how to soften them.

DIY FIXES

Invest in good skincare

Go for cosmeceutical beauty products that have higher-strength active ingredients to help minimise lines (for more on these, see page 115). Look for creams with skin-plumping hyaluronic acid, retinol to boost skin cell turnover so lines don't look so deep, and peptides to smooth wrinkles. Not smiling isn't an option!

Avoid thick foundation

Make-up that's thick, matte and powdery will settle into creases and make them look much deeper than they are. Go for a tinted moisturiser that'll help to plump them out a little or a super-light hydrating foundation. Loose powder will make them look worse, too, so avoid it at all costs. For more on this, see page 90.

DID YOU KNOW? A new treatment called Micro-Botox is very effective for getting rid of open pores on the face. It involves tiny injections all over the surface of the skin to shrink the open pores. It lasts up to four months.

AT THE CLINIC

Fillers

I started to notice my nose-to-mouth lines getting deeper when I was around 35, so I began having a little filler to plump them out. I'd recommend a very light hyaluronic acid filler such as Restylane® Vital to soften them.

Ouch factor: can be a little painful, but your doctor can apply an anaesthetic cream beforehand.

How long will it last? Up to six months.

Radiofrequency remodelling

Alternatively, try a fractional radiofrequency treatment such as Fractora, which improves the look of the whole area by tightening the skin. In the six weeks following a single treatment you will see an improvement as the skin tightens and new collagen is formed.

Ouch factor: not painful, but you may get some redness afterwards.

How long will it last? Results last up to three years.

The problem: hollow, wrinkly cheeks

When we're young our cheeks are plump and the skin is firm and springy, but over time that old enemy gravity gets to work and the fat that once gave you such pinchable cheeks slides down to become jowls. I've seen many women who went too far with weight loss and exercise in their 40s and, although they may have acquired a tiny bottom, they lost that layer of fat beneath their skin that kept their face looking plumper and more youthful, and ended up with hollow cheeks almost overnight. Here's how to keep your cheeks as plump as possible.

DIY FIXES

Don't over-exercise or crash diet

A whippet-thin figure is a tough look to pull off when you get into your late 30s and 40s, as losing too much weight makes you look drawn, and wrinkles and saggy skin look worse, too. It's important to keep your weight steady and healthy for your height and frame. Don't over-exercise or crash diet; just follow a sensible healthy eating and workout regime. For more on this, see pages 65–9.

Don't blush

Don't contour your cheeks with blush or bronzer – it'll just make hollow cheeks look even more sunken. Instead, apply a little blush to the apples of your cheeks.

Focus on your eye make-up and lip colour and try a skin-brightening base under your foundation to improve the overall radiance of your complexion. For more make-up tricks, see pages 88–96.

Help! My whole face needs a lift

Q: I'm in my late 40s and I feel as though my face is collapsing. What are the best non-surgical treatments I could have today to avoid a face-lift tomorrow? I don't relish the thought of going under the knife, but I'd like to do something to give my whole face a lift.

A: An ideal combination approach would be a Fraxel Repair laser resurfacing treatment along with a stem-cell 'face-lift' if your face needs lift as well as volume.

If it's just your skin that's looking saggy and crêpey (as opposed to problem eye bags and a double chin), then the laser alone is enough to knock ten years off your complexion – it's often called the 'laser face-lift'. It shrinks back the skin by about a third, tightening, smoothing wrinkles and diminishing age spots. You get remarkable results with this treatment but, as I've already mentioned, it's not for wimps and you'll be left with redness, flakiness and swelling for up to a week. However, your skin will continue to improve and thicken for up to six months afterwards as the deeper layers of the skin carry on healing and produce more collagen. And the results are long-lasting.

With a stem-cell 'face-lift', a doctor injects your own fat and stem cells (taken from areas where you don't want fat, such as your tummy and thighs) in the same way as a dermal filler into your jawline, across your top lip, into nose-to-mouth lines and so on.

Your stem cells help graft the fat into the area that's been injected, holding it there, so it's not broken down by the body and flushed away naturally as a dermal filler would be. It'll look good for at least five years. I've seen fantastic results with this. It not only creates volume but also feeds your skin so it looks younger and more luminous.

Change your hair

Long straight styles or hair that's too short or scraped back will emphasise hollow cheeks. Go for a style that has more volume around your face.
A short, layered bob will make your face appear fuller. I asked my friend,
celebrity hair stylist Daniel Galvin, if he had any words of wisdom on this
and he said: 'Don't go for a style that's too short as it can look severe –
particularly around the ears and the nape of the neck. If you do like a
shorter style, ask your stylist for advice on creating a cut that's softer,
fuller and will flatter your looks, ensuring it's feathered around the nape
of the neck and the jaw line to soften your features.' For more great hair
tips, see pages 83–7.

AT THE CLINIC

Sculptra®

This is an injectable volumiser that stimulates your own collagen to
smooth lines and give you a fuller, younger-looking face. It's longer-
lasting than most other injectables so bear this in mind before you opt for
it; if you don't like the results, you can't get rid of it very easily. On the
other hand, if you love how you look, it'll be great value for money. You'll
probably need three treatments a month apart.

I often recommend that patients have a little hyaluronic acid or
Novabel® filler first to see how they like it.

Ouch factor: it can be uncomfortable because there are a lot of repetitive pinpricks, but your doctor will use a topical anaesthetic.

How long will it last? Around two years.

Fat transfer

As our faces age, we lose volume in our cheeks and that full-faced, youthful look gradually disappears. Fat transfer can reverse these changes and

is now one of the most popular facial rejuvenation treatments available. It involves using a thin cannula to take fat from one part of the body, usually the abdomen, hips or thighs, and injecting it into the face. Both the area from which the fat cells are taken and the area into which they are injected will normally be numbed with local anaesthetic.

Ouch factor: can be a little uncomfortable.

How long will it last? This type of graft usually lasts about a year.

The problem: broken veins

These annoying little veins usually crop up on the cheeks, chin and around the nose, and are the result of damage to tiny blood vessels. This can be down to a variety of reasons – sun, cold weather, rosacea, damage from having too many fillers or just plain old middle age. Alcohol and spicy foods can make the problem worse.

DIY FIXES

Stage a cover-up

A really good green-tinted concealer can camouflage spidery veins by balancing out the redness. I've also found Glo Mineral Camouflage concealer in Golden or Natural works well. Alternatively, target your whole complexion with a product such as Clinique Redness Solutions Daily Protective Base SPF 15, which is a primer you apply all over your face before foundation.

Treat with creams

There are creams that can help to strengthen capillary walls. I like Medik8 Red Alert, which includes vitamin K to encourage capillary wall repair as well as botanical extracts such as bearberry and horse chestnut to soothe irritation and inflammation. I also like Avene Anti-redness Rich Moisturising Cream.

AT THE CLINIC

Laser treatment and IPL

You might need up to three sessions with lasers and intense pulsed light (IPL) before the veins disappear. The added benefit of IPL is that it has a rejuvenating effect on the skin by stimulating collagen.

Ouch factor: both treatments can be a little uncomfortable.

Lasting benefits? One to two years, although you'll need to look after your skin and protect it from the sun or you'll get new broken veins.

Sclerotherapy

Most people think of sclerotherapy as only being suitable for getting rid of visible veins on the legs, but it can also be used to treat bigger thread veins on the face. A very fine needle is used to inject a solution into the vein, which causes it to perish and disappear permanently. You might need three or four sessions a couple of weeks apart.

Ouch factor: it can sting and you should expect some bruising.

Lasting benefits? Permanent vein removal.

> **DID YOU KNOW?** The position in which you sleep can affect how your face ages. If you sleep on your side you'll get more wrinkles on your cheeks, while sleeping on your front can give you a wrinkly forehead. The best position is on your back. This isn't a natural position for a lot of people (me included), but try putting pillows by your sides to stop you rolling over.

The problem: age spots

Age spots (also known as liver spots or sun spots) are a common form of hyperpigmentation – where patches of skin become darker than the rest of your complexion. They're caused by that old enemy sun damage. Pigment-producing cells deep in the skin, called melanocytes, are stimulated by sunlight to produce more pigment to protect us from the sun, and sometimes they can go a bit crazy and overproduce. The result is patches of darker skin that look like dirty marks – lovely!

The single most important thing you can do to prevent age spots – and I know I sound like a broken record – is never bake in the sun and wear face cream with an SPF of at least 15 on your face all year round.

DIY FIXES

Lightening creams

Once the damage has been done, ZO Brightenex™ is my product of choice to zap age spots. It targets all four stages of skin discolouration by inhibiting melanin formulation and minimising existing pigmentation.

A word of warning: I think it's best to avoid other 'lightening' products, as I don't know any that work without being toxic. You might find creams on the Internet containing kojic acid – a mushroom derivative, which has been used for thousands of years in Japan as a skin lightener – but this is about to be banned in the UK. It can be toxic in very high doses and there have been cases of people using large quantities to lighten their skin.

Creams containing hydroquinone – a chemical that destroys pigment-making cells – are only available on prescription from your doctor. Hydroquinone can't be used for long periods of time or on larger areas of skin as it produces a carcinogen, but it's safe and effective in low doses and in small amounts.

AT THE CLINIC

Intense pulsed light

Although laser treatment works well for age spots, I think IPL is probably the most effective clinic treatment for getting rid of them. It's more suited to paler skins. It'll take a couple of weeks for the age spots to fade and, over time, they will darken again so it's vital to stay out of the sun and use a sunscreen. IPL will also improve the condition of your skin, making it firmer and smoother. I'd recommend having between four and six sessions. Remember, you mustn't have it when you have a suntan as the light could damage the surrounding skin.

Ouch factor: it can hurt!

How long will it last? Up to 18 months, but it can be permanent if you treat your skin properly and use sunscreen. We often give our patients Lumixyl™ after a treatment to help prevent age spots returning.

Peels

Peels literally peel off those surface layers of dead skin, revealing newer skin beneath. I'd recommend going for a glycolic acid peel to fade age spots, although it won't get rid of them altogether. It will also improve your complexion overall, boosting radiance and making skin feel smoother. And if you have a course of treatments over several months, your skin will also start to firm up because it's producing more collagen.

Peels will only do a certain amount, though, so if you have stubborn age spots, I'd recommend laser resurfacing, which is very effective at reversing sun damage and stimulating new collagen. But I'd suggest starting off with light peels to see how you get on, particularly if it's your first clinic treatment.

Ouch factor: it depends which peel you have. A light peel will be slightly tingly, whereas a deeper one will hurt! See page 167 for my easy guide to working out which peel might be right for you.

All you need to know about peels

When you have a chemical peel, your doctor or therapist will cleanse your face thoroughly then paint on the peel and leave for the required time. Afterwards, your skin is cleansed again and moisturiser is applied. Here's the lowdown on the four main types of peel and what you can expect from each one:

- Glyclolic acid peel – my favourite. This acid occurs naturally in sugar cane and gently dissolves the glue-like substance that holds dead skin cells on the surface of your skin. It comes in a variety of strengths – from a salon strength of 20–40% to a medical version of 70–90%, which must only be administered by a cosmetic doctor. It's good for freshening up a tired, jaded complexion, smoothing fine lines and is suitable for all skin types – even sensitive. You'll need a course of six to get good results, then a top-up once a month. You'll only experience a mild tingling that tails off after a minute or two and there's no downtime.

- Jessner peel – a medium-strength peel that can deal with more damage than glycolic acid. It combines resorcinol, lactic acid and salicylic acid for deeper exfoliation. It's good for diminishing acne scars, sun damage and wrinkles, and also decreases oil production. Let's be honest: this peel burns like hell. You may be reduced to tears, depending on your pain threshold. Your skin will peel and flake for about seven days afterwards until the newer, smoother skin is revealed.

- TCA peel (trichloroacetic acid) – comes from the acid that gives vinegar its pungent taste and smell. It's a medium-to-deep peel that's used in concentrations of 10–35% and is pretty painful. Your skin blanches (frosts and turns white). It works well on some skins to remove acne scars, hyperpigmentation and fine lines, although it's not suitable for darker skins. Between one and three treatments a month apart are recommended and you'll need up to a week to recover while your skin is red and flaking.

- Amelan multi-mask peel – uses an acid that's found in Japanese sake and shiitake mushrooms and is effective on skin with pigmentation problems following pregnancy or sun damage. It also refines pores and smoothes fine lines. You'll only need a day to recover. Most clinics would prescribe a skin lightening cream afterwards to help prevent the pigmentation returning. This is slightly tingly, but not painful.

How long will it last? After one treatment you'll see the benefits for around a week, but a course of six will give you fresher skin for between six and twelve months.

The problem: double chins and jowls

When you think about ageing, the chin probably isn't the first thing that springs to mind, but this area is prone to several nasties, from a deepening chin wrinkle and enlarged pores (both of which can be easily fixed with a little Botox) to harder-to-treat problems such as double chins and jowls. A double chin is often caused by weight gain and/or ageing, but it can also be a genetic characteristic – take a look at your parents to see if it could be in store for you! Unfortunately, it's just one of those areas where fat likes to find a home as we get older. Jowls are those really unattractive little pockets that hang down either side of your chin and are the result of fat from your cheeks sliding down over the years. Not something to look forward to! Here's what you can do to reverse the damage and help prevent it, too.

Can you get a 'no-knife face-lift' with Botox alone?

Q: I'm 37 and just starting to notice the first signs of wrinkles and sagging. I've thought about having Botox, but I'm young and want to look as natural as possible and be able to move my face. What would you suggest?

A: At our clinic we've developed a treatment called Microtox, which is the sort of technique that could be right for you. Other clinics will also offer more subtle treatments like this, so do ask. We use a botulinum toxin called Azzalure® and inject smaller amounts than would be used in regular Botox treatments to give the whole face a lift. You'll need more injections than a regular treatment, but the needle is tiny so you'll hardly feel it.

You'll have a series of injections into those areas that are showing signs of ageing – along the jawline, around the lips and eyes, between the eyebrows and high on the forehead – which gently tightens and lifts skin, shrinks pores, erases spider veins and softens lines.

Personally, I think the results are fantastic and look very natural. You'll still have movement and no one would ever guess you'd had a treatment. It'll look like you've been on the holiday of a lifetime!

DIY FIXES

Manage your weight

The first thing to do is lose weight if you need to and start introducing healthier foods to your diet. That means more fruit, veg, high-fibre carbs, lean white meat and fish – and less red meat, full-fat dairy products, processed foods, fatty and sugary snacks.

Watch out for alcohol and fizzy drinks in particular, which often cause puffiness around your face and neck. For more on this, see pages 63–5.

A facial exercise for double chins

Exercising your face regularly can help give you a tighter jawline. Try this one: sit up straight and tilt your head back so you're looking at the ceiling. Keep your lips closed. Next, make your lips round, as if saying the letter 'O', and hold for a count of 20, then relax and bring your head back to the normal position. Finally, slap under your chin with the back of your hand for a couple of minutes. Aim to do this two or three times every day.

Facial exercises for jowls

Once jowls have settled in, no amount of exercise is going to shift them, but you can help prevent them by working your facial muscles regularly. Here are a few exercises to try:

- Smile slightly, then squeeze your lips so they're tightly closed, flexing your neck muscles. Hold for a few seconds, then keep repeating for about a minute. Do this once a day.
- Sit up straight and lean your head backwards so you're looking up at the ceiling. Let your mouth relax so it's open. Next, stick out your tongue and try to touch your chin with the tip of your tongue. Keep your tongue in this position for a few seconds, then pull it back in. Repeat five times. Do this once a day.

- Try the 'shovel' exercise. Sit up straight, then lift your lo
  up over your top lip and slide it down again. Repeat 12 t.
  times, three times a day.
- Try an exaggerated closed-lip smile – you should feel those
  muscles working!

Chew gum

Yes, chewing gum regularly can help tighten your jaw muscles. Make sure it's sugar-free, though, as a nice tight jawline won't be much good if your teeth are rotten.

AT THE CLINIC

Radiofrequency remodelling

This can help double chins and jowls by tightening the skin and dispersing fat, but the result will depend on how much fat or sag you have there. If it's not too much, you'll probably be pleased with the results.
Ouch factor: a hot sensation while you're having the treatment, but not painful. You may experience a little pain and redness afterwards.
How long will it last? A couple of years.

> **TIP!** I'd never recommend regular liposuction for the chin and neck area as it's far too aggressive, but SmartLipo is a great alternative for small- or medium-sized pockets of fat and it's minimally invasive. See page 184.

The problem: marionette lines

Marionette lines are the ones that run from the corners of your mouth down to your chin. This problem is also known as puppet mouth, although I like to call it miserable mouth syndrome. In terms of DIY fixes, sadly there isn't much you can do to banish or camouflage these grooves. Good anti-ageing skincare can help to make them look a little less obvious. Avoid thick foundations and loose powders, which will settle into the lines to make them look worse. To fix them, these lines need some filling in at the clinic.

AT THE CLINIC

Fillers and other injectables

Hyaluronic acid-based fillers such as Restylane® work well to soften marionette lines, while other injectables such as Sculptra® and Novabel® can plump them out and will last longer. A more permanent option would be to have your own fat and stem cells (taken from your thighs or tummy) injected into these lines, but it's a pricier option.

Ouch factor: a pinching or burning sensation with the injections.

How long will it last? About six months for hyaluronic acid fillers, between one and two years for Sculptra® and Novabel®. If you go for injections of your own fat, it'll age naturally with your body.

The problem: neck wrinkles and crêpey skin

The neck is often the area that gives away your age, but it's amazing how many women stop their beauty regimes at their chin. Their necks never see moisturiser, let alone sun protection. The skin here is delicate and exposed to the elements daily so you need to treat it exactly as you would the skin on your face. That means exfoliating, moisturising every day with an SPF cream and treating it regularly to other face savers such as masks, peels and anti-ageing serums. Crêpey, wrinkly skin and the dreaded turkey neck are all perils of getting older, so it pays to get into the habit of treating this area with tender loving care as early as possible.

DIY FIXES

Treat it to good anti-ageing creams

You can buy special neck-firming creams – see page 125 – but my advice is simply to use good anti-ageing facial products, which will do the job just as well. Go for facial washes, exfoliators and creams that contain rejuvenating AHAs such as glycolic acid to improve the texture and firmness of your skin. The Jan Marini Skin Care Management System™ has good glycolic acid products from cleansers to creams and serums. It's particularly important to wear an SPF if you use glycolic products to protect your skin from sun damage.

Peel away the years

Glycolic acid at-home peels are good for sloughing off those surface layers of dead skin cells and tightening the skin, too. Simply apply the solution, leave for the required time, then wash off with a cloth. My favourite is NeoStrata Citriate Home Skin Peel.

AT THE CLINIC

Botox, fillers and peels

Tiny amounts of Botox (see page 149) can soften necklace lines (those horizontal bands you get when you bend your neck) and vertical lines that start under your chin and travel towards your collarbone. It'll last for up to four months, so you'll need regular top-ups. Very light hyaluronic fillers such as Restylane® Vital can be used (see page 159), but the skin on your neck is so fine there's a risk that the fillers could look lumpy and obvious. For crêpey, sun-damaged skin, a course of light glycolic peels (see page 167) can improve texture and help to even out skin tone.

The problem: turkey neck

Unfortunately, there are no DIY tricks that will get rid of this loose skin on your neck once it's there but, to help avoid it, keep your weight steady as you can develop turkey neck after dropping a few dress sizes. Stay out of the sun to protect the fine skin on your neck and always cover up with a high SPF cream.

DIY FIXES

Facial exercises
These can improve the muscle tone in the neck. Here's one to try:
• Sit up straight and tilt your head back so you're looking at the ceiling. Keep your mouth closed and relaxed. Next, move your lower lip over your top lip as far as possible and hold for a count of 10. Relax and repeat 10 times.

AT THE CLINIC

Thermage
If the problem isn't too bad, this radiofrequency treatment can tighten the skin and put energy into the deep layers of the skin to produce

collagen, making skin thicker. It's worth considering as a preventive measure in your early 40s when you see the beginnings of a problem. The results take up to six months to show, but they're good when they arrive! **Ouch factor:** it's an uncomfortable treatment rather than painful as it puts a lot of heat into the skin. I'm a wimp and I could cope with it, especially after I saw the results on other people.

How long will it last? Several years.

Fraxel Repair laser

If the problem is more advanced, you could opt for Fraxel Repair. It hurts, but it is effective at shrinking back the skin in this area.

Ouch factor: expect swelling, bruises, bumps and redness for a week or two while skin is peeling. Definitely painful, but I'd say it's worth it.

How long will it last? Several years.

Unfortunately, if you have lots of hanging, loose skin the only thing for it is a surgical neck lift. See pages 182–6 for Nip Tuck options.

Complexion boosters that work

If injectables or peels aren't your cup of tea and you don't feel ready to brave laser resurfacing treatment, these face-saving treatments can give your skin a rejuvenating boost.

AT THE CLINIC

Cosmetic acupuncture

This treatment can have a great effect on your face if you have regular sessions. Tiny needles are inserted into acupuncture points on your face to lift specific areas, improve skin tone, boost blood flow, soften lines and reduce puffiness and eye bags. Don't expect dramatic results after one session – the effects are cumulative – but it's a good 'maintenance' treatment. The needles don't hurt and you should leave feeling relaxed and with a real sense of wellbeing. Can't be bad! See page 178 for advice on how to find a practitioner in your area.

The MLD facial

Any facial massage treatment is a good idea because it boosts circulation and improves muscle tone, but my personal favourite is manual lymphatic drainage (MLD). It's great for relieving puffiness in the face and neck and stimulates your lymphatic system to work more efficiently to get rid of waste and toxins from tissue. It also improves skin tone and firmness, leaving your complexion revitalised. A nice treat, too. See page 281 for contact details to find a massage therapist in your area.

TIP! Try this DIY facial massage. Place your fingers on either side of your neck right under your ears, then gently move the skin in a downward motion towards the back of your neck. Repeat 10 times, gradually moving your fingers down and further away from your ears. Next, place your fingers on top of your shoulders, either side of your neck, and gently massage by bringing the skin closer to your collarbone. Repeat the shoulder massage action five times.

Salt microdermabrasion

This is a far less aggressive form of microdermabrasion, which traditionally uses aluminium crystals. It's like a gentle sandblasting of the skin to remove the dead skin cells that make complexions dull and flat. One session will leave your skin super-smooth and radiant, but I'd recommend an initial course of six treatments a couple of weeks apart. If you have them regularly, they'll help soften lines and improve skin texture and tone. My clients love this treatment. It's a nice lunchtime fix before an evening event.

Micro-needling

A-listers are queuing up for this facial in Hollywood. It's a little more hardcore than the facials you'll be used to, but it gets great results. First of all your skin is cleansed, a peptide serum is massaged in, then a barrel-like hand roller with hundreds of very fine needles is rolled over your skin leaving tiny pinpricks (there can be a little bleeding here and there). This activates a wound-healing response to stimulate collagen, which in turn thickens ageing skin. Anti-ageing peptides are also able to penetrate deep into the skin.

It's an uncomfortable treatment, rather than painful. After one session your skin will look plump and dewier, but I'd recommend a course of six every two to three weeks. The natural healing process lasts for several months in which time your skin will carry on improving.

THE NEW ANTI-AGEING FACIALS

These days there are all sorts of weird and wonderful facial treatments aimed at making your complexion more youthful. Here are a few of my favourite ingredients to help hold back the clock.

Nightingale droppings

Yep, you read that right! We have a treatment at our clinic called the Geisha Facial based on the ancient Japanese use of nightingale droppings. These contain uric acid, which is known for its cleansing and nourishing benefits. The droppings are powdered, sanitised and mixed with aromatherapy oils to make a mask, which we leave on for 20 minutes. Afterwards skin looks smooth, luminous and plumped up.

Whale sperm

You read that right, too! We have a Spermine Facial that uses whale sperm and salmon egg extract for a tighter, firmer, more radiant complexion. It's a great quick fix for tired, lacklustre skin.

Enzymes

At our clinic we've developed a facial using an enzyme from the green papaya that digests dead skin cells without harming healthy, living cells. Because these enzymes are selective, they're less harsh than traditional exfoliators. Thirty minutes later a fresher, younger-looking complexion will be yours! To get the benefits at home, try Jan Marini Skin Zyme Mask.

Finding a good practitioner

For all non-surgical clinic procedures, always go to a properly qualified cosmetic doctor who specialises in the treatments in question. You might think that's obvious, but it worries me that such a cavalier attitude is taken to some procedures, especially Botox. At one point there was a trend for Botox parties where the wine would be flowing and a doctor would whizz over and inject all the women at the party. Someone's living room is not the right place to have Botox! Your medical history should be taken during a proper consultation in a controlled environment. It's an invasive procedure – a toxin is being injected – so it's not something to giggle over with friends between glasses of wine.

Never let a beauty therapist give you Botox or fillers, because they don't have enough understanding of facial anatomy. I'm a very experienced therapist, but I would never attempt to administer these treatments. A light peel can be done by a beauty therapist, but she must have training from the company that supplies the peels and should have a training certificate for insurance purposes – ask to see it.

Can salon facials turn back the clock?

Q: Are there any good beauty salon facials that have a significant anti-ageing effect? Or would I be best spending my money on a stronger clinic treatment that's proven to get results?

A: Salon facials have come a long way in recent years and there are some really good ones, but I feel the greatest benefit with the majority of them is the relaxation factor. They're fantastic for a deep cleanse and to hydrate your skin but any wrinkle-smoothing or 'lifting' effects will be temporary.

When choosing a facial, the most important thing is to look for one that offers massage as part of the treatment, as this really is beneficial. It stimulates the circulation to bring blood to the surface with much-needed nutrients and helps to flush out toxins. It also increases skin elasticity, loosens scar tissue on acne sufferers and improves sebaceous secretion to moisturise the skin, improving its condition and texture overall.

Rather than opt for an incredibly expensive 'anti-wrinkle' salon facial, start with a good deep cleanse and skin-feeding treatment such as Dermalogica's Multi Vitamin Facial, which leaves skin feeling nicely plumped up.

I'm also a fan of Elemis facials; their Tri-Enzyme Resurfacing Facial targets superficial lines, scarring, blemishes and uneven skin tone and is good for a smoother, more radiant complexion. I also like their Visible Brilliance Facial as it uses micro-circulatory massage.

Some beauty salons have a doctor or nurse attached so they can provide certain non-surgical treatments such as Botox, but I would always choose a medical aesthetic clinic, staffed by doctors and therapists.

A clinic like this won't usually provide the fluffy, relaxing salon treatments. It's foremost a medical environment that focuses on injectables, lasers and peels, treatments for skin conditions such as acne, rosacea, hyperpigmentation and scarring, as well as body procedures including liposuction. Doctors will be able to prescribe any medication that may be needed to work alongside topical treatments.

DO YOUR RESEARCH

When it comes to finding a doctor, a personal recommendation is always a good option. The trouble is, many women only tell their mother or their best friend because they don't want people to find out what they're having done. In my experience, a lot of women don't even tell their husbands.

You'll find medical aesthetic clinics in most big cities – check your local phone book for ones in your area or look online. Maybe your GP will be able to recommend a doctor or clinic. But it's worth doing some research on the Internet and looking at press articles to find out which doctor consistently comes out top for the procedure you want. In my opinion it's worth travelling to another town to consult a doctor who has a good track record for the procedure you're after.

There's a growing trend for travelling abroad to specialist skin clinics but I'd strongly advise against this. What happens if something goes wrong? And unfortunately, sometimes it does. You may get an infection that requires attention or you may need advice if you're not recovering in the way you'd expected. After-care is vital – sometimes for up to three months after a surgical procedure. I'm not saying overseas clinics aren't good – some may be excellent – but they are not accessible once you return home, so you have very little back-up.

And be wary of adverts in the back of magazines. These may prompt you to think about having a procedure done, but look into the clinics and doctors properly in the way I've described before committing to anything. Just because you see a lot of advertisements for a clinic doesn't necessarily mean it's good.

THE INITIAL CONSULTATION

Make sure you feel comfortable enough with your doctor to talk honestly about what you want – and what you don't want. If you don't feel happy, go and see someone else. You can always ask for the doctor's GMC (General Medical Council) number to check their qualifications if you feel unsure. You could also ask to speak to a patient of theirs who's had the treatment you're considering and look at their before and after pictures (with their agreement, of course). A reputable doctor will usually have plenty of patients willing to sing their praises.

Ask yourself if you like the staff at the clinic. Are they helpful? Is the doctor polite to them? Is the clinic clean and tidy? Can you get an appointment immediately? It isn't a good sign if the waiting room is empty and you can be scheduled for the procedure the next day. Unless you're lucky enough to get a last-minute cancellation, expect to wait a couple of weeks to see a good aesthetic medical practitioner.

When you go for your consultation, I think it's a good idea to take along a photograph of yourself when you felt you looked your very best. This isn't so they can try to replicate it (that's never going to happen), but it'll give them an idea of how your face used to be and the kind of look you're after.

Finally, be aware that even if you choose the best doctor in the world, there's always a risk that something could go wrong or that you simply won't like the results. Unfortunately, this is the chance you take with any procedure, so try to be realistic about your expectations and prepared for the fact that things might not turn out as you'd hoped. Consider this carefully before embarking on any procedure, be it non-invasive or surgical.

Nip tuck know how

Sometimes surgery is the only option but I believe it should only be considered as a last resort, when nothing else will work. This may sound odd considering that I am married to a plastic surgeon, but I know he agrees with me. As more and more treatments are developed to help us avoid surgery, I believe that over the next ten years we will see fewer and fewer people taking this route. There are several reasons for this. We all have busy lives and don't want to have a month to six weeks' downtime after an op. Surgery can also be very expensive. There's an overnight stay to pay for as well as an anaesthetist and a surgeon. After some ops, you can be left with terrible scarring, so you're just swapping one problem for another. You have to work out which problem you'd rather have, or ask yourself if you could improve the problem by 30 to 40% with a non-surgical treatment.

However unhappy you are with a particular part of your face or body, before you rush headlong into surgery my advice would be to start with the least invasive option and work your way up. For some problems, non-surgical options are much more successful. For example, a face-lift doesn't put volume back into your skin to mimic the plumpness of a youthful complexion in the way that treatments such as Sculptra® or even laser resurfacing can. It simply stretches it tight.

If you start anti-ageing treatments early – say in your late 30s or early 40s when you first start noticing changes – then you may not have to go down the surgical route later. Having said all that, there are some problems that no lasers or injectables will solve. And it's good to know what's available so you can make an informed choice. I firmly believe in the right treatment for each individual – the one that suits their problem, lifestyle and budget.

THE MOST POPULAR ANTI-AGEING SURGICAL TREATMENTS FOR THE FACE

FaceTite, the newest no-knife facial rejuvenator

FaceTite, a minimally invasive treatment, is the most advanced facial tightening procedure available and gives an instant lift to saggy skin around the eyes and on the forehead, cheeks, mouth and jowls. The procedure uses radiofrequency and involves inserting a fine probe into the fatty layer just under the skin, causing the skin to warm and tighten. FaceTite tightens skin by up to 40 per cent, despite being much less invasive than other treatments that achieve similar results.

Ouch factor: minimally painful as the procedure is performed under a local anaesthetic, but there will be some swelling and bruising for about seven to ten days after the procedure.

How long will it last? Within a few minutes you will have much tighter skin that looks and feels better. Then, as new collagen is produced over the following three to six weeks, you will see a continuous improvement, with the final results visible 12 weeks post procedure. Results will last up to five years, similar to a mini face lift, then the skin will age naturally, depending on your genetics and lifestyle.

Blepharoplasty for droopy eyelids and bags

Eye bags are common in middle age, but if they're an inherited characteristic you can develop them in your early 30s. I would always recommend getting eye bags removed sooner rather than later. They can put ten or 15 years on your face and, once they've settled in, they're not going anywhere!

Surgery will remove the excess fat and skin from under the eyes through an incision below your lower lashes. The op is also used to remove excess skin from the upper eyelids that give people a droopy, hang-dog expression.

Downtime: it's a relatively minor op that's performed under local or general anaesthetic, but it usually takes a couple of weeks to recover and for the swelling and bruising to go down.

Laserlipolysis for double chin and jowls

My preferred technique is SmartLipo, which is only slightly invasive and requires a local anaesthetic. A 1mm cannula is inserted just under the surface of the skin through a tiny incision, then a very small laser heats up fat cells, which burst, allowing the fat to be gently sucked out. The laser also cleverly tightens skin so you're not left with any sag.

Downtime: it's been termed 'lunch-hour lipo' because it's a quick procedure and people have been known to go straight back to work afterwards, but I'd recommend taking it easy for a day or two.

Neck lifts for loose skin

For some people with a bad case of turkey neck, where skin is hanging loose, a surgical neck lift might be the only option. Incisions are made in the lower hairline or behind the ears, the skin is pulled up, the excess is removed and it's stitched into place.

Downtime: the scars will be firm and pink for at least six weeks and may remain the same size for several months. They could take up to two years to fade so you won't be able to wear your hair up without them being seen.

There is also a ribbon lift for necks, where an absorbable ribbon implant to lift and secure the neck tissues is inserted through a short incision around the earlobe. It is passed from below the earlobe to the back of the neck just below the jawline. The ribbon is then pulled back to lift the neck and define the jawline, and secured to the deep tissue behind the ear. This lifting action produces excess skin around the earlobe which is trimmed to complete the procedure. The implant anchors the tissue during the normal healing phase and is absorbed by the body after ten to twelve weeks.

Downtime: you'll be out of action for about two weeks with bruising.

Brow lifts for droopy, wrinkly foreheads

These will raise your eyebrows, lift skin that hangs over the eyes and smooth forehead lines. The most usual method these days is a technique called an endoscopic brow lift, in which the surgery is performed through tiny cuts in your hairline, so there's minimal scarring.

There's also an internal brow lift, where the brow is lifted through a cut in the crease of the upper eyelid skin, so no scars can be seen.

In my view, you should avoid a coronal brow lift. This involves an incision across the top of your scalp, hidden within your hair. Through the cut, the surgeon removes excess skin, shortens the muscles that cause frown lines and lifts your eyebrows. Ouch! It's an outdated method, will leave you needing silly haircuts and these days there is just no need for it.

Downtime: each method requires either a local anaesthetic with sedation or a general. You will usually be able to go home the same day and you should be back to normal within two weeks.

Mid face-lift to lift sag

Face-lifts are rapidly becoming an outdated concept, but for people in late middle age for whom things have gone too far, a surgical procedure might be the only way to make a difference. A mid face-lift removes lower eye bags and lifts saggy cheeks that make nose-to-mouth furrows much deeper. An endoscope (a tiny camera-like device) is inserted through small, deep incisions in the muscles of the face to view the procedure internally. The surgeon adjusts the fat and muscle tissue, pulling up the middle of the face to smooth and tighten the skin. The cuts are then stitched.

Traditionally, access to the cheeks and lower eyelids is by using an incision hidden in the lower lash line and sometimes an incision in the nose to mouth lines. This technique is best for people who are drooping and need to be lifted upwards, rather than horizontally or diagonally.

A more dramatic technique involves making incisions in the temples, hidden behind the hairline. This gives the surgeon access points through which he can lift facial muscles and skin both vertically and diagonally. **Downtime:** up to four weeks and expect swelling and bruising. Big ouch!

TIP! For more information on cosmetic surgery and to find a surgeon, contact the British Association of Aesthetic Plastic Surgeons on 020 7430 1840 or visit their website (see page 281). All the advice given on pages 178–81 for finding a good practitioner applies to plastic surgeons as well as cosmetic doctors. In particular, I wouldn't recommend travelling overseas for surgery. It may be cheaper, but it will be much harder to go for follow-up consultations and advice.

seven
Make the Most of Your Assets

I know from the women I see in my clinic that most of us are obsessed with the shape and size of our breasts. This is backed up by the latest figures that show breast augmentation is the most popular cosmetic surgery procedure in the UK today.

The fact is, there is nothing that can make you feel sexier than having a perky bust, which is why from the moment we develop breasts we agonise over how they look. Are they too big? Too small? Too droopy?

At the age of 16 I was embarrassed by my tiny boobs, as all my friends seemed to have bazookas! But as I got older, I developed my own double D cups, and I loathed the attention they got.

Our issues with our breasts only get worse as we get older, thanks to a number of age-related problems that occur in this area. I'm talking about crêpey skin, age spots, breast fold lines, drooping and loss of cleavage. Not surprisingly, these changes can leave you feeling far from sexy. It's no wonder that over the years many of us become unhappy with our breasts and decide to do something about it. Fortunately, there are a lot of methods short of surgery to keep this area looking younger for longer. So, if you want to achieve an ageless décolletage, read on.

The problem: crêpey skin

The skin on the décolletage is very delicate and particularly prone to photo-ageing. Years of sun damage combined with the natural thinning of the fat layer under the skin, leads to thinner skin, which looks as though it has no 'give' to it, plus the dreaded age spots and a crêpey, leathery texture. But help is at hand. Here are some proven ways to tackle the problem.

DIY FIXES

Smooth things out

You should give your neck and cleavage the same level of attention and care you lavish on your face. When applying your regular cleanser and moisturiser, take them right down to your chest. Always apply in an upwards movement to avoid dragging down the delicate skin.

It's very important to keep the décolletage hydrated as it doesn't produce as much natural oil as the skin on your face. Look for creams that contain retinol (a type of vitamin A), AHAs and antioxidant vitamins; these will all help to smooth and brighten the ultra-delicate skin in this area. I like Jan Marini C-ESTA® Hand and Body Cream, which is rich in vitamin C.

Polish away the years

Just as on your face, a build-up of dead cells can make the skin on your chest look dull and lifeless. Restore the flush of youth to your décolletage with regular, gentle exfoliation. Sloughing away those dead cells that make lines and wrinkles appear deeper will give skin a much more radiant appearance.

> **TIP!** There's no need to run out to buy an expensive exfoliator – just look in your larder. A handful of sugar mixed with a couple of teaspoons of honey will create a fabulous, gentle scrub.

Stay safe in the sun

We often expose the delicate skin of our décolletage to the elements in plunging necklines – in summer and winter – so don't forget to protect this area from photo-ageing. Remember that prevention is always better than cure. Make sure you apply a sunscreen of at least SPF 15 all over this delicate area whenever it's on show, come rain, snow or shine!

AT THE CLINIC

Microdermabrasion

This treatment is fabulous for refreshing the top layer of your chest skin and treating age-related problems such as sun damage, superficial age spots and fine lines. My favourite version is Naturepeel, which uses salt to sandblast the skin and is very gentle. Dead skin cells are exfoliated away, revealing fresher, more radiant skin underneath. This is a great treatment to have in the run-up to a wedding or other special occasion where you want to flash a little flesh. For the best results I'd recommend between three and six treatments a week apart, followed by a monthly top-up session.

Ouch factor: just a gentle tingling and no recovery time.

How long will it last? You will notice a difference after the first treatment, but a course will get the best results. After that you'll need regular top-ups to maintain the effects.

Intense pulsed light (IPL)

To up your game a little you could try photorejuvenation, using IPL. This treatment can clear up age spots, improve skin tone and smooth the appearance of crêpey skin and I've seen some impressive results on this area of the body. An intense flash of light is aimed at your décolletage, which releases energy into the skin. It targets sun damage and triggers your natural healing process, which encourages collagen production for younger-looking skin.

Ouch factor: yes, it can hurt, but it's over fairly quickly.

How long will it last? You'll need four to six treatments, but the results should last from a year to 18 months.

Light to medium peels

The great thing about using a peel on your décolletage is that you don't need an industrial-strength acid to see results. The skin here is so delicate that anything from a mild glycolic acid peel to a stronger TCA peel will work wonders, by removing dead skin cells and fading sun damage and wrinkles.

Ouch factor: tingling for glycolic, but TCA is like having red hot chilli peppers on your skin.

How long will it last? A couple of weeks, but you can maintain the results with a good skin cream containing AHAs. Afterwards you must wear an SPF to protect the newer skin from the sun and help prevent age spots reappearing.

Mesotherapy

This can be a good way to boost the health of the skin on your décolletage. A series of tiny micro-injections delivers a special vitamin formula into the skin. I think some of the rejuvenating effects of this treatment are caused by your body's healing response to all the pin-pricks, which stimulates collagen.

You will be left red and pinpricked for a few days afterwards, so this is not an emergency 'night before the party' treatment, but after a course of about four sessions you will see a significant improvement in the condition of your skin. I'd recommend between three and six treatments, depending on your skin, each one two weeks apart.

Ouch factor: any injection is going to sting, but as the needle is very tiny, there's only a little discomfort.

How long will it last? The results will last about a year and after that you'll need a yearly top-up of between one and three treatments.

PRP (platelet rich plasma) or biogel rejuvenation

This innovative treatment uses injections of platelets and powerful growth factors, taken from your own blood, and is especially effective for crêpey skin. Platelets contain substances called growth factors that encourage the production of collagen and generation of new capillaries to rejuvenate the skin and eliminate wrinkles.

Ouch factor: only what you'd expect from any injection, but a topical anaesthetic should be applied first so it's not painful.

How long will it last? It's a permanent repair and will age naturally with you. Lasts up to ten years.

Laser micro-peel

Laser resurfacing is my favourite way to treat sun-damaged crêpey skin – on the face or body. In a micro-peel, a Smartxide laser is used to puncture thousands of tiny holes into the surface of the skin, stimulating the natural production of collagen, to repair the tissue. Your skin will look thicker and ten years younger within weeks.

Ouch factor: a mild burning sensation.

How long will it last? Up to three years.

Laser resurfacing with CO$_2$ lasers

This isn't for the faint hearted! An ablative CO$_2$ laser, Fraxel Repair, works in much the same way as Smartxide, but it's a deeper and more aggressive treatment. The laser penetrates deep into the skin to stimulate your body's natural healing process and the production of collagen. The surface of your skin will be red for a week or so after but then feel softer, brighter and have a more even tone, and it will continue to improve for three to six months after the treatment.

Ouch factor: this is painful, but the pain vanishes when the procedure is completed.

How long will it last? Up to ten years.

The problem: breast fold lines

Yet another of the annoying changes that occur as the years pass is that the thin supporting muscles under the chest skin become weaker and thinner, resulting in a drooping effect and causing vertical lines to develop between your breasts. At first these lines are only noticeable when you get up in the morning, fading as the day goes on. However, over time they gradually become more severe until they're a permanent fixture on your neckline. But don't panic – here's my advice on banishing these blemishes.

DIY FIXES

Sleep on your back

One of the biggest chest crinklers is the way we sleep. Curling up on your side means that by the time morning comes around your chest will be covered in creases, like a crumpled-up shirt. One solution is to retrain yourself to sleep flat on your back. Investing in a c-shaped curved pillow (sometimes called a 'geisha pillow') can help stop you rolling over on to your side.

Get some nightly support

Special bras that you wear in bed can stop the formation of chest creases and soften any that you already have. La Decollette is one such bra that provides a layer of cushioning between the breasts to prevent them being squeezed together while you sleep.

Try a super serum

A skin serum is a good night-time treatment to help soften chest lines, as the light texture doesn't overload this delicate area of skin. Look for one with firming ingredients that contains retinol for maximum anti-ageing benefits. CCLIFT (available from my Harley Street Clinic – see page 277) is good for this.

AT THE CLINIC

Micro-needle therapy

Micro-needling is a great treatment to give your cleavage skin a smoother finish and help eliminate fine lines. A drum-shaped instrument covered in tiny micro-needles is rolled over the area to be treated, stimulating collagen formation. See also page 177.

Ouch factor: slight discomfort, but not painful. A topical anaesthetic will be applied to numb the area before treatment.

How long will it last? Up to a year.

Botox

Just as it works to smooth out facial lines, Botox can help soften unsightly chest wrinkles in some cases. See also page 150.

Ouch factor: as with any injection it will sting, but the needle is very fine and a cooling device is used on the skin to keep discomfort to a minimum. **How long will it last?** About four to six months.

Restylane® Vital

This is a wonderful treatment for rehydrating and restoring volume to the skin. Tiny amounts of thin hyaluronic acid dermal fillers are injected just under the skin to instantly smooth out lines and wrinkles. You will need up to three treatments over a period of two weeks.

Ouch factor: local anaesthetic cream is applied to the area to minimise any discomfort.

How long will it last? About a year, but you'll need annual top-up treatments to maintain the effect.

The problem: droopy boobs

All breasts sag as we get older; whether you're big-breasted or small, gravity wins in the end. Weight loss, childbirth and breast-feeding make the situation worse, I'm afraid. And while the bulk of the damage is done with your first child, it gets progressively worse with each subsequent pregnancy.

As the breasts start to droop, the nipple position will slide. This is because the rectus abdominus muscles under the breasts become stronger over time and you lose volume at the top of the breast, so nipples droop. Unfortunately, we tend to exercise these muscles inadvertently in everyday movements such as sitting down and getting up from a lying down position.

But breasts that point south aren't something we have to just grin and bear; here are my top fixes for a perkier pair.

DIY FIXES

Get fitted for an instant lift

It's a fact that most women in this country wear a bra that's completely the wrong size for them, leading to a saggy bust and lots of unsightly bulges. A good bra can make you look years younger. Get measured for a bra that fits you properly and gives you good support. Stores such as M&S and Debenhams offer free bra-fitting services.

Strap them in!

In terms of prevention, there is no better investment than a good sports bra. Your breasts are supported by fragile ligaments, which are not elastic, so once they are stretched they cannot snap back again. During exercise your breasts bounce and pull on these ligaments, causing them to stretch and this leads to sagging boobs. Make sure your breasts are properly supported before any physical activity.

Pad things out

Tucking a couple of gel pads or 'chicken fillets', as they've become known, inside your bra can work wonders for small boobs that need to be perked up. They lift your breasts to create cleavage where once there was none. You can also buy gel-filled bras which have the same effect and mean you don't run the risk of losing a pad on the dance floor! Try Ultimo for gel-filled styles.

Work it out

As with any muscle, the pectoral muscles above the breasts can become weak unless exercised regularly, resulting in saggy boobs. For firm pectorals, try palm pushes. Stretch your arms out in front of your chest and press your palms together hard. Hold for five seconds, relax and repeat ten times. Chanting 'I must, I must, I must improve my bust!' is optional.

Bust-lifting creams

No lotion is capable of lifting your breasts. If only! However, a good firming lotion can help improve the appearance of sagging skin to boost the overall look of the area. Mama Mio do a marvellous product called Boob Tube Bust and Neck Firmer, which many beauty editors have dubbed a 'Wonderbra in a jar'. I wouldn't go that far, but it contains a good moisturising mixture of nourishing Omega oils and shea butter (which holds moisture in the skin), along with CoQ10 to boost collagen.

TIP! Don't sit with your arms under your breasts supporting them – it will only highlight the fact that you have a wrinkly cleavage. Take a look in the mirror to see what I mean. Yuck!

AT THE CLINIC

Botox

As well as ironing out lines on your forehead and your décolletage, this muscle-relaxing toxin can also give sagging breasts a lift. Muscles work in pairs. If one set is damaged, its partner will overcompensate. Injecting Botox into the pectoral minor muscles beneath the breasts will weaken them, causing the major muscles to rise, giving your breasts a lift in the process. Clever, eh?

Ouch factor: it will sting.

How long will it last? About four to six months.

Laser skin lift

A Fraxel Repair CO_2 laser can shrink sagging skin to give a lift to the breasts – but the procedure isn't ideal for everyone. It's better suited for women with smaller breasts with only a mild to moderate droop, as treating the skin alone won't be enough to lift heavier breasts.

Ouch factor: a feeling of heat, which can be uncomfortable.

How long will it last? Up to two years if you use sun protection.

Fillers

A thick, hyaluronic acid filler called Macrolane™ can restore lost volume to breasts and give your cleavage a much-needed lift. Also known as the 'Boob Jab', Macrolane™ is injected deep into the breast tissue using a thick needle. The only down side is that it can make nipple droop worse.

Ouch factor: local anaesthetic will be used to numb your breasts, so you won't feel any pain during the procedure, but they will be slightly bruised and swollen for a few days afterwards.

How long will it last? A year, then it will need to be topped up.

Fat transfer injections

How many times have you looked in the mirror and wished you could have the fat on your hips relocated to your breasts? Well, guess what? You can! Fat can be taken from your waist, hips or buttocks, using micro-liposuction, and injected into the breasts to fill them out.

Ouch factor: some pressure and stinging can be felt while fat is removed and again when it is injected into the new area, but it is rarely seriously painful.

How long will it last? About a year, but results are variable and your breasts may need further treatment to rebalance them after 12 weeks.

The laser bra lift

This new and promising technique uses a CO_2 laser on the surface tissue layer of the breasts to create a boosting effect. It punches thousands of tiny holes into the skin, triggering the skin to produce extra collagen to heal itself. The extra collagen produced makes the skin thicker and therefore restores elasticity, giving the breast a lift and some extra oomph.

It's great for women who are worried about having a full-on breast-lift op. You should expect some initial swelling, and the skin will peel and flake for about a week, but you'll be back to normal activities after two weeks. Women with very heavy breasts won't benefit from this treatment, though.
Ouch factor: performed with a local anaesthetic and sedation. You should expect a little discomfort during the procedure.
How long will it last? Up to five years, and the effects will age with you.

The problem: boobs that are too big

Never happy, are we? If we have small breasts, we use padding to make them bigger and if they are larger, we want to minimise them. But the truth is, as we get older, big boobs can make us look matronly and overweight, cause back problems, and lead to all kinds of nightmares when choosing clothes. Plus, of course, the larger the breast, the bigger the droop. So it's no surprise we need a bit of help using the following techniques.

DIY FIXES

Don't try to minimise
Minimiser bras are designed for larger bust sizes (DD upwards) and aim to make big boobs look smaller. But in my experience, they can actually

> **TIP!** It's much more important to get a well-fitted bra, which holds your breasts in, rather than a minimiser that straps them down. Aim for a smooth look, with your nipples level with halfway between the elbow and armpit.

make you look worse – especially if they don't fit properly. They can create a solid ridge and have half your bosom spilling out over the top of the bra cup. Another danger area is under the arms. It looks and feels awful when you have bra spam bulging out of the side of your bra.

Fashion tricks

You can easily dress down your ample assets. Avoid high necks, round necks and halter necks. And steer clear of scarves and boxy jackets, which just draw attention to them. Also, don't be tempted to hide yourself under floaty fabric, as anything baggy will make boobs look larger.

V-neck, scoop and sweetheart necklines are more flattering for us busty ladies. Anything that keeps our breasts in line while separating them is a good option, so wrap dresses are a great day-to-evening staple. For more on dressing for your shape, see pages 101–9.

> **TIP!** There's no point in spending a fortune on underwear, clothes and treatments if what you really need is to lose a little weight. A healthy diet and exercise plan can help you drop a couple of bra sizes, with no surgery required.

AT THE CLINIC

At the moment there are no clinic treatments to minimise breasts, so the only option for smaller breasts is a breast reduction operation (see page 201).

Nip tuck know how

More than 8,000 breast augmentations are performed in the UK each year, and this trend looks set to continue, as the numbers continue to rise steadily year on year.

What is set to change, however, is the manner in which we boost our busts. I'm pretty sure that implants will soon be a thing of the past, as we opt for healthier, more natural forms of enhancement, such as stem cell-enriched fat grafts. These have the added benefit of avoiding the stigma attached to silicone implants, as you'll be able to say quite truthfully that your breasts are all natural!

Similarly, there are some interesting new developments in the area of boob lifts. As with all types of plastic surgery, though, I would urge you to think of it as a last resort if you are deeply unhappy with your current shape.

THE MOST POPULAR SURGICAL TREATMENTS FOR BREASTS

Breast implants

In this classic op, implants (usually silicone) are inserted under the breast tissue, and sometimes under the muscle, through incisions made around the nipple, under the breast or under the armpit. With implants, it's important not to go too big for your frame. If they're too big, they'll be heavy and get droopy – less is more.

Downtime: you will have to spend one or two nights in hospital, and you'll need to take at least ten days off work. There could be some swelling for up to three months and in some cases you won't be able to lift your arms above your head for up to six weeks. There will always be some scarring, but it can fade over time.

TIP! Trial-run bigger boobs before going under the knife, by buying a bra the cup size you would like to be, then pad it out and see if you like how it feels.

Breast reduction

With a reduction, excess breast tissue, fat and skin are removed through an anchor-shaped incision that circles the areola (pink area around the nipple), extends down in a vertical line and follows the natural curve of the crease beneath the breast. The nipples are then repositioned higher on the breast.

Downtime: you may only be required to stay in hospital for one night, and will be able to return to work within a fortnight. You will have to wear a surgical bra 24 hrs a day for one to two weeks while the swelling and bruising subside. Scarring may take months or sometimes a year to settle.

TIP! Speak to your GP to see if you qualify for breast reduction on the NHS. The surgery is only available if your breasts are causing significant health problems, such as back or neck pain, and not for cosmetic reasons alone. For more information, visit www.nhs.uk/conditions/breast-reduction.

Breast lift

The ultimate fix for sagging breasts is uplift surgery. Three incisions, which form an anchor shape, will be made in your breasts, to enable the surgeon to remove excess skin and move the nipple to a higher position, before closing the incisions with dissolvable stitches. However, you will be left with extensive scarring, so while you will look great in clothes, your breasts will not look their best naked.

Downtime: you'll be hospitalised for a couple of nights. You should take at least two weeks off work and wear a supportive sports bra for a couple of months.

The latest development – the invisible bra

This is a new technique that's good for women whose breasts have sagged due to weight loss. Unlike a traditional breast lift, where the breast is held up with skin alone, this technique uses a mesh material called Breform™ that's shaped like a bra cup. This cup or cone is placed underneath the skin and attached with stitches to the layer of fat above the breast tissue under general anaesthetic. With time, your body produces a fibrous tissue that holds the cup in place, like an internal bra. It provides support without putting any strain on the scars or the skin, so it's unlikely your breasts will sag again.

You'll be left with the same scars as a regular breast lift and, as with other breast enhancement surgery, there is quite a big ouch factor.

Because this treatment is so new some doctors have expressed concern that the long-term risks are unknown, but Breform™ has been used safely in hernia operations for 40 years.

Downtime: as with breast augmentation, you'll need a couple of weeks off work and your breasts may be painful for a few weeks after surgery.

eight
Sexy Arms and Younger-looking Hands

Until a few years ago I didn't give my upper arms a second thought. I'd go shopping for gorgeous sleeveless cocktail dresses and never worry about the need to cover up batwings. I didn't have any, right?

Then I went on holiday and caught a glimpse of a blubbery upper arm in the mirror as I was walking to the pool bar one day to get an ice cream. 'Is that *my* upper arm?' I wondered, doing a quick double-take. 'Oh my god, no ice cream for me, thanks, just a mineral water!'

My arms had suddenly morphed into somebody else's. When did that happen? Almost as soon as my plane hit the tarmac back in London, I hit the gym. 'Exercise, exercise, exercise,' was my mantra. Even at home I never missed an opportunity to try to tighten my bingo wings. I used whatever came to hand as weights: cans of baked beans, bottles of water, cartons of milk, you name it – but to no avail. It seems in my case it was a bit too late in the day for a new exercise regime to give me the toned, sculpted arms I lusted after. That's when I started exploring the other options, which I describe below.

We're more aware when our hands begin to age because we see them every day and can spot the warning signs of dryness and crêpey skin. On pages 209–15, I'll give you my best tips on keeping your hands looking fresh and young-looking.

The problem: wobbly, crêpey, bumpy upper arms

At the clinic I see women of all ages who hate their upper arms – even girls in their 30s complain about them. It's just one of those areas women are sensitive about. Some claim they were born with chunky arms. For others, weight gain causes the extra blubber, and in some cases weight loss leaves saggy skin behind. Then there's plain old age to blame for wobbly, crêpey skin and cellulite.

There's always the option of three-quarter-length sleeves, cardies and shrugs to cover up the problem (for more on this, see page 106). But if you're not ready to give up on your arms just yet, read on.

DIY FIXES

Tone up the wobble

If the problem isn't too advanced, exercise can make a big difference to muscle definition in your arms, but you have to do it religiously. I'd say you need to squeeze it into your day at least three times a week. The following exercises are easy to do at home and you can build up to more repetitions as your strength increases.

- Bicep curls target the muscles at the front of your arms. Pick up some hand weights from any sports shop – around 2kg is a good starting weight, and you can buy heavier ones as your strength increases. Either stand with your feet shoulder-width apart or sit on a chair in an upright position. Hold a weight in each hand and let your arms hang by your sides, palms facing forward. Keeping your elbows close to your sides, curl the dumbbells up towards your shoulders in a slow, smooth movement. Uncurl slowly back to the starting position. Aim for two sets of 12 repetitions three times a week.

> **TIP!** Resistance bands are great for toning your arms and a good alternative to hand weights when you're travelling. These bands or tubes of rubber (some with handles) are cheap, lightweight and portable. Once you have some, there's no excuse for not fitting in that workout, wherever you are.

- Tricep dips target the muscles at the backs of your arms that give you those nasty bingo wings when they start to droop. Put a sturdy chair against a wall and sit on it, then grip the edge of the chair so your knuckles are facing forwards. Your knees should be bent and your feet on the floor, hip-width apart. Slowly lower your bottom down in front of the chair, bending your elbows until your upper arms are parallel to the floor. Slowly and smoothly bring yourself back to the starting position with your arms straight and your bottom level with the seat. Aim for two sets of 12 repetitions, three times a week.
- Push-ups target the triceps and shoulder muscles. Many women swear by this exercise for firming up flabby arms. Lie on your tummy with your elbows tucked into your sides and palms flat on the floor. Keep your knees on the floor as you push up. Make sure your back is straight, your tummy muscles are pulled in and your head is in line with your spine. Slowly lower yourself so your chest

touches the floor, then push up again. Don't straighten your elbows when you come up; keep them slightly bent. Aim for two sets of eight to 12 repetitions, three times a week. As you get stronger, you can try a full push-up where you lift your whole body off the floor, balancing on your toes.

TIP! Jennifer Aniston and Geri Halliwell are among the celebs rumoured to keep their arms toned and sexy by using a Kettlebell. This exercise gadget looks like a cannonball with a handle and it gives arms (and the rest of your body for that matter) a really intense workout when you swing it in a variety of different moves. For stockists, see page 279.

Be a smoothie

The skin on your upper arms can become dry, crêpey and bumpy. Get into the habit of exfoliating your arms every other day in the shower, using a gentle body scrub to get the circulation flowing and slough off flaky skin. Afterwards, treat them to some super-hydrating body cream. If you keep up this routine, you'll soon notice the difference in the quality of your skin, which should feel smoother and plumper.

TIP! For a really effective at-home exfoliation treatment, soak a flannel in hot water, wring it out well then briskly rub over your upper arms several times. Next, massage a home-made mix of coarse sea salt and olive oil into your skin and remove with the warm flannel. Finally, use a dry flannel and rub briskly till your skin is dry.

Little white bumps

Keratosis pilaris is the name for those rough white bumps on the outer upper arm area, which are caused by a build up of dead skin. You can keep them under control by using an exfoliating cleanser daily, such as my own Harley Street Skin Body Buffer, followed by a cream with AHAs to dissolve the glue-like substance that holds the dead skin on the surface. I like NeoStrata's Daytime Smoothing Cream. Or try a microdermabrasion product intended for your face as a special treatment once in a while. We have one at our clinic (Harley Street Skin Microdermabrasion With Pearls And Diamonds) that uses crushed diamonds to remove dead skin. It also contains lactic acid, so your skin feels super-smooth afterwards. It would be too pricey to use a product like this on your arms very often, but it's a good little beauty boost if you're wearing a sleeveless dress for a special event.

Ditch the orange peel

Cellulite loves to collect on your upper arms – not such a problem in winter when you can bury them in layers of clothes, but a big issue when summer comes around and you have to put them on display. As we all know, once the dreaded orange-peel skin has settled in, it's a nightmare to get rid of. No cellulite cream is going to cure the problem, but it can have a temporary firming and smoothing effect on your skin so lumps and bumps are less obvious. It's worth a try if you have the extra cash to splash out on something other than a bog-standard body lotion – just don't expect dramatic results! (For more on this, see page 129.)

For a less expensive approach, try dry skin brushing your upper arms regularly with a natural bristle brush. I've met women who swear by body brushing to reduce the appearance of cellulite. Brush upwards from your hands towards your heart, using long, firm strokes. The theory is that brushing boosts the lymphatic system, speeding up the elimination of toxins. It'll also get rid of the build-up of dead skin cells to reveal fresher, more radiant skin. It's best to do it before a shower.

AT THE CLINIC

Massage
Salon or clinic massage treatments are good for circulation and can help to reduce the appearance of cellulite if you have them regularly. A manual lymphatic drainage massage (MLD) is particularly beneficial as it encourages the removal of waste and toxins from body tissue.

Light peels
If you're willing to throw some money at the problem, a chemical peel using glycolic acid will remove dead skin cells and improve the texture of the skin on your upper arms. It'll even out skin tone, fade sun damage and leave your arms feeling super-soft. If you're considering this option, I'd go for a whole body peel for a real feelgood boost.
Ouch factor: gentle tingling.
How long will it last? A couple of weeks, but you can maintain the results with a good cream containing AHAs.

Reaction
Reaction is the latest treatment designed to tighten and smooth the skin, improve its elasticity and refine its texture, while also helping to reduce cellulite. Treatment incorporates radiofrequency to break down fat with vacuum therapy to stimulate lymphatic drainage, and this combination initiates three different processes: deep tissue heating,

mechanical stretch and mechanical massage. The procedure takes about an hour and I'd recommend a course of six to eight treatments, each a week apart.

Ouch factor: there is no downtime and it's not painful, although some women might find it a little uncomfortable.

How long will it last? With yearly top-ups, results will be permanent.

> **TIP!** There's no point spending your hard-earned cash on a treatment like Reaction only to continue with the bad lifestyle habits that contribute to the build-up of cellulite. Cut back on junk food, eat lots of fresh fruit and veg, drink plenty of water and stay active to maintain a healthy weight. For more cellulite-busting tips and treatments, see pages 234–40.

The problem: age spots and crêpey skin on the hands

They say you can tell a woman's true age by her hands and, I have to say, if I'm not sure I always take a quick glance. I remember being scolded by my mother for sitting at my great grandmother's feet, pulling up the skin on her hands and counting how long it took to settle back into place. Goodness, I must have been an awful child – but it shows I was interested in skin even then! Try this yourself: if the skin springs back immediately, it's in good shape, but if it takes a few seconds to reshape, you're in trouble.

Our hands take a battering. They're constantly exposed to the elements and are in and out of water all day long. We lose the fat in our hands as we age due to hormonal changes and the skin becomes thinner so veins look more prominent. Couple this with a few age spots and it's bad news. No matter how beautifully your nails are painted, it won't detract from scrawny, witchy hands!

It pays to give your hands a little more attention. Like a lot of things, you don't always appreciate what you have till it's on its way out or gone altogether. But it's not all doom and gloom – there are ways to tackle this little group of horrors. Here's how.

DIY FIXES

Protect hands from the sun

First things first. I know I'm always going on about the importance of sun protection, but it really is vital if you want to keep your hands looking youthful, as they're subjected to the weather all year round. Wear a hand cream or sun lotion with SPF 15 in winter and go up to SPF 30 in the warmer months. I know we all feel better with a suntan but please fake instead of bake! I'm a big fan of BeautyLab Peptide Tanning, which stimulates melanin production, giving you a really natural colour and, compared to most other fake tans, it smells pretty good, too.

For more on faking it, see pages 45–8.

DID YOU KNOW? You need to protect your hands from the sun even when you're driving as those ageing UVA rays can penetrate glass.

Moisturise, moisturise, moisturise!

To help keep dry, crêpey skin at bay, get into the habit of using hand cream regularly. Well-hydrated skin always looks younger and plumper.

Keep a tube of hand cream somewhere handy, so you remember to apply it a few times a day. This might be on your desk at work, by the sink at home or pop a travel-sized tube in your handbag. I keep my hand cream in the car door and every time I get into the car, I put some on.

Three of my favourite hand creams

- Vaseline Intensive Rescue Soothing Hand Cream
  I love this product – it's such a bargain, but it works a treat to lock in moisture, keep skin really soft and protect it from the elements.
- NeoStrata Hand & Nail Cream
  I'm a huge fan of this brand. As well as being super-moisturising, this cream includes a polyhydroxy acid (PHA) to target the signs of ageing.
- Jan Marini Age Intervention Hands
  This is the most powerful hand cream I've ever used and a personal favourite. It contains acids to tackle crêpey skin and lightening agents to reduce sun damage. It also has SPF 15.

TIP! For maximum hydration, apply hand cream to the back of one hand, then place the backs of your hands together and rub around in a circular motion. This way you don't waste the cream on the palms of your hands and the moisture is getting to where it's needed most.

Give your hands a 'facial'

If your hands are in dire need of some TLC, treat them to a 'facial' once a week. First wash them with a moisturising soap that won't dry them out, then exfoliate the backs of your hands. You can buy special hand scrubs but I prefer to use a gentle facial exfoliator that includes AHAs to slough off dead skin cells. Why buy two products if you only need one that can multi-task? You could also use a little body scrub – just don't rub too hard. Now apply a hydrating face mask and leave for a few minutes to let it work its magic. Rinse off and finish with some nourishing hand cream.

For an extra treat, do this routine before going to bed. Slather on loads of hand cream then pop on some cotton gloves. The next morning when you take the gloves off your hands will be incredibly soft. This is perfect for very dry, cracked winter hands.

Rubbing in some glycolic acid serum a couple of times a week will also help to improve the texture of your skin and plump it up over time by stimulating collagen.

For tips on younger-looking nails, see pages 98–100.

TIP! For an easy home-made hand scrub that really works, add a handful of oats to ¼ cup of water until it's absorbed. Next, add a tablespoon of lemon juice and a teaspoon of olive oil. Rub the mixture into your hands and leave for a few minutes. Rinse with warm water and pat dry.

Fade away

Hands are prone to age spots from sun damage and they're not easy to shift once you've got them. One product I've found works wonders at fading these unsightly brown marks is ZO Melamin™. Just make sure you use it with an SPF 15 to prevent age spots from returning.

AT THE CLINIC

Glycolic peels

A course of six glycolic peels can freshen up the skin on your hands, reduce hyperpigmentation and stimulate cell turnover to reveal newer, plumper skin. It's not a miracle cure, but you'll definitely see an improvement. Afterwards you must wear an SPF to protect the newer skin from the sun and help prevent age spots reappearing.

Intense pulsed light (IPL)

This is a gold-standard treatment for erasing age spots. The light beams break up pigment and the age spots dry up and peel off within a couple of weeks. Use an SPF 30 afterwards to protect your hands.

Ouch factor: yes, it can hurt.

How long will it last? Around 18 months.

Laser resurfacing

This treatment goes deeper than IPL. The intense heat from the laser stimulates the formation of new collagen and also causes the outer layers of the skin to peel away, giving the hands a smoother, firmer, more youthful appearance. I've had this treatment and the results are excellent – definitely worth putting up with a little ouch factor! Depending on the depth of the treatment it can take anything from five days to two weeks to recover. It's very important to keep your skin well hydrated with an emollient cream and sun protection afterwards.

Ouch factor: yes, it can hurt, but a topical anaesthetic cream will be applied to your hands about 30 minutes before the treatment.

How long will it last? Up to three years if you exfoliate regularly and wear sunscreen.

The problem: veiny hands

There's nothing like prominent veins to make your hands look very 'old lady'. I've noticed that women who work out a lot tend to have incredibly veiny hands. It's because they have very little body fat, so the veins stand out on their hands where the skin is thinner. In terms of DIY tricks for veins, there isn't a lot you can do, but here are some suggestions.

DIY FIXES

Cheat no. 1: use make-up

A good tip that celebrities use for red carpet events is to wear make-up on their hands. This helps cover up blue veins as well as other blemishes, so hands appear smoother and younger. I like to use mineral make-up as it provides good coverage, is easy to apply because it's a powder, and it doesn't rub off on your clothes. It also has a natural SPF of 20 so it's good for daytime, too.

Cheat no. 2: wear gloves

If you have no time, no cash, or simply don't fancy going the treatment route, get yourself some gloves. They're an easy cheat in winter, and you could buy fingerless lace evening gloves or long satin Audrey Hepburn-style ones for a glamorous event.

AT THE CLINIC

Sculptra®

This clever volumising product can be injected between the veins to stimulate collagen production, replacing tissue where the fat has been lost. You'll need three or four treatments a month apart.

Ouch factor: this can be uncomfortable, but your doctor will use a topical anaesthetic 30 or 40 minutes before the treatment. Expect your hands to look red and spotty for a day or two afterwards.

How long will it last? Two to three years.

Restylane® Vital

This fine hyaluronic acid can be injected superficially all over the hands to plump them up. It works well for some people. I'd recommend three treatments, two weeks apart.

Ouch factor: your doctor will apply a topical anaesthetic 30 minutes before the treatment. Your hands should feel back to normal the next day.

How long will it last? About a year.

Nip tuck know how

As with all other cosmetic surgery procedures, I'd advise trying the non-surgical options first. But if your arms or hands really bother you and you've got the money to spare, here's my lowdown on the operations you can have.

THE MOST POPULAR SURGICAL TREATMENTS FOR ARMS AND HANDS

SmartLipo to reduce batwings

This is a minimally invasive procedure that works on the upper arms. It's nowhere near as aggressive as liposuction and it requires only a local anaesthetic. A laser is inserted through a tiny incision into the fat layer, then the fat is melted and gently sucked out through a tiny cannula. The laser also heats the skin, which stimulates collagen production. That nasty lumpy fat is permanently removed and, if your skin hasn't been too damaged by the sun, it can tighten nicely.

Downtime: you can get back to your normal routine the same day, but expect bruising and swelling for a week or two.

Brachioplasty for saggy arms

This is the op that's used to remove excess skin and tissue under the arms. An incision is made from your armpit to your elbow, so the scarring is quite extreme. I personally can't see the point of going through a general anaesthetic for this, as the scarring means you probably wouldn't want to show off your arms anyway. If you're considering this option, think long and hard about whether the benefits outweigh the scarring.

Downtime: you can't lift anything heavy for about four weeks, and swelling and bruising take between two and four weeks to heal well. It can be six months before scars start to fade.

Fat transfer for scrawny hands

In this procedure fat is taken from your tummy, hips or thighs (where most of us are carrying a little excess baggage), then injected into your hands in the same way a filler would be. It's all done under a local anaesthetic. The effect lasts about a year, so you'd need to repeat annually to maintain the appearance.

Downtime: it takes about two weeks to recover.

Cell-enriched fat transfer for scrawny hands

The difference between this and regular fat transfer is that the fat taken from your tummy, hips or thighs is processed with your own stem cells before being replaced. This means it'll have a blood supply keeping the fat alive so it's able to graft on to your hands. This procedure will cost you more but it's permanent so you won't need to return for top-up treatments.

Downtime: around two weeks, as with regular fat transfer.

nine

A More Youthful Midriff, Back and Bottom

I remember the days when I used to run out of the shower past the full-length mirror with only a tiny towel protecting my modesty and think nothing of it. Then one morning when I was sitting on the bed wrapped in my tiny towel I noticed a little tummy flab poking out. Where on earth had that come from and why hadn't I noticed it arriving? It's scary how these things creep up on us. One minute you're on the beach in a string bikini, the next your hormones have gone crazy and your waist has disappeared.

It's not fair. As your face gets thinner and you discover cheekbones you didn't know you had, your waist gets thicker due to fluctuating hormone levels. This normally starts happening in your late 40s. It's as if your body starts revolting against you and slams on the metabolic brakes, causing you to lay down fat around your hips and midriff. Then there are love handles (they sound a lot sweeter than they look), back fat, bra spam (where fat spills over the straps and under the arms) – and did I mention loose, crêpey skin, stretch marks and a flat, saggy mum bum? And you thought crow's feet were the biggest age giveaway.

what can you do? You can sit around telling yourself that you're more interesting than ever, so it doesn't matter if you have a muffin top. Or you can try some of the ways described in this chapter to turn back time on your body.

The problem: mummy tummy and midriff bulge

Weight gain or loss and pregnancy (which causes the abdominal muscles to separate) can dramatically change the way your stomach looks. I know many women who lost their baby weight quite quickly, but could never get rid of that little pot belly and just learned to live with it. As we age and our metabolism slows down, fat naturally wants to deposit itself on our lower body, including the hips and tummy. You don't have to put up with it if you don't want to, though. Follow my tummy-taming tips and tricks.

DIY FIXES

Tone up

Pilates is great for this area because it's all about strengthening the core muscles – the deeper muscles in your abdomen and back. The exercises are also good for improving posture and there's nothing like slumped posture to make a mummy tummy stand out more. Here are a few easy at-home moves to firm up your tummy and tone your waist:

- Sit-ups for a flatter, firmer tummy – Start by lying on the floor, with your legs hip width apart, knees bent and feet flat on the floor. Cross your arms over your chest so your hands are on opposite shoulders, or interlace your hands behind your head with your elbows out to the sides, in your peripheral vision. Keep the weight of your head in your hands and take care not to pull your neck when doing this move.

- Breathe in to prepare, and as you breathe out, engage your tummy muscles by drawing your belly button in towards your spine, slowly nod your chin to your chest, and curl your shoulders off the floor. Keep the tailbone down and hips soft, curling up about halfway. Make sure you maintain the gentle curve in your lower spine and don't imprint the lower spine into the floor. Hold for a few seconds, breathing in, then curl back down on your out breath, keeping your belly engaged. Repeat five times if you're a beginner – you can always build up to doing more as your strength increases.
- Once you've built up to 20 sit-ups over a couple of weeks, take the exercise a little further to really whittle your waist. Start the sit-up as usual but, when you come up, twist your waist by rotating your ribcage across to one hip. Keep the chest open, and make sure the movement comes from your waist rather than your shoulders or elbows to really make the abdominals work. Then twist across to the opposite side. Repeat to each side 5 times, and when you have more strength build up to 10 times either side. (Make sure you don't hold your breath: move on the out breath and return to the start on the in breath.) Believe me ladies, this is the one move that really makes a difference to my waistline and all it costs is a little sweat (and maybe a few tears!).

TIP! A really easy way to get a flatter stomach is to repeatedly hold your tummy in. Simply pull your belly button in towards your spine and hold for a few seconds. It works the **transversus abdominis**, the muscle that helps pull in your tummy. Do it anywhere, any time!

- Torso twists for a trimmer waistline – stand up straight with feet shoulder-width apart and slowly twist to one side, then the other, keeping your hips facing forwards. For a bit extra, hold a stability ball or a pair of dumbbells out in front of you.

TIP! Still got an old hula hoop in the loft? Dig it out and start spinning to tone up your waistline.

Dress smart

Figure-fixing underwear with tummy control panels or waist-cinching all-in-ones will help to give your waistline a smoother silhouette under clothes. Try www.figleaves.com for a wide range of shapewear.

Help define a thick waist with tailored dresses or use a wide belt over tunic tops and dresses to nip you in. Don't try to cover up in baggy styles! Flatten a tummy with trousers and skirts that sit just above the hips – and go for flat-fronted styles instead of pleats or anything with lots of volume as these styles will just make you look bigger.

For more on dressing for your shape, see pages 101–9.

Improve the quality of your skin

Every time you bathe or shower, apply a nourishing body cream to hydrate the skin on your tummy so it looks smoother, softer and younger. My advice would be to look for a lotion with CoQ10 – one of my favourites is NeoStrata Bionic Lotion 15 PHA, which is great for dry, crêpey skin and exfoliates gently, too.

AT THE CLINIC

Reaction

I've mentioned Reaction, a non-invasive and painless treatment, in relation to dimply upper arms, and it has the same benefits for wobbly tums and bottoms. The machine uses radiofrequency and vacuum therapy to help smooth and tighten skin.

Ouch factor: there is no downtime and it's not painful, although some women might find it a little uncomfortable.

How long will it last? With yearly top-ups, results will be permanent.

BodyJet™

Another treatment that works wonders on wobbly tummies is BodyJet™, a minimally invasive treatment that removes fat instantly. A variation on traditional liposuction, this is a water-jet-assisted procedure that washes away the fat without damaging blood vessels or nerves.

Ouch factor: slightly uncomfortable, but treatment uses local anaesthetic and there is little recovery time.

How long will it last? Results are permanent.

The problem: stretch marks

Stretch marks are horrible and, although they can crop up on other areas of the body such as the breasts and thighs when the tissue tears due to weight gain or a growth spurt, the most common place for them to appear is on the tummy during pregnancy. Some women go through several pregnancies and never get a hint of a stretch mark, while others aren't so lucky. It depends on what type of skin you have, your age (if you're older, skin doesn't have the same bounce-back ability) and how big your bump is. And while you'd never trade in your little angels for a blemish-free belly, these marks can get you down. They certainly don't make you feel sexy and bikinis are out (for tips on beachwear, see page 108). In the meantime, here are a few things you can do.

DIY FIXES

Massage in a special oil or cream

This can help prevent stretch marks developing and diminish the appearance of existing ones by improving the elasticity of your skin. My favourite products are:

- Bio-Oil
- Elemis Japanese Camellia Oil
- Revitol Stretch Mark Prevention Cream

All are safe to use during pregnancy and, for the best results, you should apply them twice a day in a circular motion.

AT THE CLINIC

Dermaroller™ therapy

This procedure, called microneedling, is rapidly becoming one of the most requested anti-ageing treatments and is hugely popular with celebrities in the UK and in Hollywood. I love it because it is simple yet very effective and far less invasive than lasers or surgery. There is hardly any downtime following treatment and it is about as natural as you can get – perfect for those who want something that works but is non-surgical. A barrel-like hand roller, called a Dermaroller, with hundreds of very fine needles, thinner than your own hair, is rolled over the skin, leaving tiny pinpricks. This is perceived by the body as damage, which activates a wound healing response to regenerate the skin, boosting collagen levels, which in turn thickens fine, ageing skin and helps treat stretch marks and other skin damage. For best results, I would recommend a course of six treatments, each two to three weeks apart.

Ouch factor: uncomfortable rather than painful.

How long will it last? It will take a few months for the results to appear fully and then the effects will be permanent.

For more dramatic results for stretch marks, see stem cell-enriched fat transfer, page 230.

The problem: back fat and bra bulges

That nasty fat that bulges out over the sides of the bra under your arms and around the straps is a menace to many of us. It's due to weight gain that creeps up on us with age, but it can alter the shape of your breasts and looks horrible under close-fitting tops – particularly around your back. Then there's the fat that settles around our lower back in the form of 'love handles', which often bulge over the top of your jeans. Yuck!

Here are some ideas to banish those lumps and bumps.

DIY FIXES

Lose pounds if you have to

If you need to reduce your overall body fat, this is good a place to start. You don't have to turn into a gym junkie overnight, but try building more fat-burning activities into your life – brisk walking, dancing, swimming, cycling. It helps you stay motivated if it's fun, too. For more on this, see page 67.

Try the back squeeze

This move works your mid and upper back muscles, toning them for a sexier look. It'll also work your arms and shoulders a little, too. Start by sitting on the floor with your legs straight in front of you. Place the middle of a resistance band against the soles of your feet and grab each end of it. Wind it around your hands once if you need to, so it's taut when you're sitting in an upright position. Pull your elbows back, squeezing your back muscles and keeping your elbows close to your body. Return to the starting position. Aim for two sets of eight to ten repetitions – you'll feel it the next day if you've done it correctly. If you did this five times a week, you'd also improve your posture and reduce the risk of back and neck ache.

Get a bra that fits you

Most women wear the wrong bra size – and an ill-fitting bra can make you bulge in all the wrong places. Some women look as though they have an extra set of boobs on their back! Get measured at a department store.

Treat your back to some TLC

The skin on our backs is neglected because we can't reach it to apply exfoliator or body cream. I always think that if you're going to pay for a salon or spa treatment, you should choose something that includes your back, which otherwise gets no attention. Some spas will offer special back treatments with exfoliation, masks and massage to target specific problems such as spots or crêpey skin. At home, use a long-handled body brush and work upwards towards your shoulders to help get rid of dry skin and boost circulation. Jump in the shower, then get your other half to smooth on some nourishing cream on those hard-to-reach bits. At the clinic, a course of light glycolic peels is a good option for smoother, younger skin.

I bet many of you will be surprised by your real bra size. Go for styles with wide straps and three hooks on the clasp as these offer more support and you're less likely to get flesh bulging over the edges. Shoestring straps are only for skinny minnies with A-cup breasts!

Don't be clingy

If it's a smooth silhouette you're after, banish all clingy fabrics from your wardrobe – they'll highlight even the tiniest bulge. Natural fabrics such as cotton or silk won't cling and are much more flattering than anything synthetic. When it comes to your lower back bulge, look for trousers and jeans with waistbands that sit above your hips to hold in any wobbly love handles, and go for a full brief that won't allow anything to escape over the top.

AT THE CLINIC

Reaction

Just as Reaction can work wonders on cellulite or mummy tummies, it can also help to remove excess back fat. See page 208 for more information.

Ouch factor: there is no downtime and it's not painful, although some women may find it a little uncomfortable.

How long will it last? With yearly top-ups, results will be permanent.

The all-over body peel

A body peel is probably one of the most luxurious treatments that you can have and great for giving you an all-over glow. Chemical peels, usually a combination of alpha hydroxy acids (AHAs), remove dead skin and improve the texture of the skin. Many brides request one of these peels at our clinic a few days before their big day, and A-listers love to pop in for one before a red carpet event.

First you have a shower using an exfoliating wash, then you dry off thoroughly. A prepping solution is applied to 'degrease' the skin then the peel will be applied to each area separately. It is washed off with tepid water, a neutraliser is applied and washed off, then a moisturiser with SPF is applied. It takes about an hour, but you should be left with more even skin tone and your body should feel soft and smooth. I'd advise using a light moisturising cream with AHAs in it on a daily basis to help maintain the results.

Ouch factor: slight tingling.

How long will it last? Skin looks fresher for around a week after one session.

The problem: saggy bottom

Just as our breasts head south with age, our bottoms follow suit, giving us a saggy, flat behind that's sometimes referred to as a 'mum bum' – the exact opposite of a nice pert, peachy little butt. We spend years of our lives complaining that our bums are too big, then one day we wake up and realise those once-round, firm cheeks are getting more deflated by the day. Yep, we are never happy! If it's dimples and wobble that worry you, turn to pages 234–40, where you'll find loads of tips and treatments for beating the dreaded cellulite. But if it's sag that concerns you, here's how not to be a droopy drawers.

DIY FIXES

Work those butt cheeks!

- Buttock clenches are the easiest way to firm up those muscles. What's more, you can do this exercise literally anywhere, even standing in line at the supermarket (so long as you're not wearing skin-tight clothing). Simply stand with your feet hip-width apart and clench your bottom muscles, hold for a few seconds and repeat for one or two minutes.

- Lunges are also good – stand up straight then lunge forward slowly with one leg, so the shin of your back leg is parallel to the floor and you're balancing on the toes of your back foot. Return slowly to the starting position and repeat on the other leg. Make sure your front knee doesn't go past the tips of your toes. Aim for two sets of eight to ten repetitions.
- Next try squats – stand with your feet shoulder-width apart and slowly lower your body as if you're about to sit on a chair, until your thighs are parallel with the floor. Hold for a moment then slowly return to your starting position. Try to keep your weight in the heels. Aim for two sets of eight to ten repetitions.

You'll start to see a difference if you do these three exercises for five minutes each day.

Cheat your way to a more shapely rear

There are pants that will make your bottom appear more pert and curvacious. Try Huit, Just A Kiss Padded Shorty, which has firm foam padding in the rear to give the droopiest of derrières a lift.

Beware of crash diets

Drastic diets are the enemy because you lose muscle as well as fat, which can lead to that 'loose' look. We need strong muscles to keep good shape, but when the body is 'starved' it holds on to its fat stores and uses lean tissue and muscle for energy instead.

Look after your skin

Massage, body brushing and regular exfoliation will all help improve the appearance of the skin on your bottom, giving it a smoother, younger look.

They'll also boost circulation, bringing much-needed nutrients and oxygen to the skin. If you can bear it, a little DIY hydrotherapy with the shower hose can help keep skin tight – simply blast your bottom with alternating jets of hot and cold water. That'll wake you up in the morning!

AT THE CLINIC

Botox

I bet you didn't imagine you could have Botox in your bottom! In this case it's nothing to do with relaxing wrinkles. Your doctor will inject into the skin just below the buttocks, which relaxes the 'pull down' muscles and allows the 'pull up' muscles to work more easily. You'll notice a difference after a few days.

Ouch factor: not really.

How long will it last? Between four and six months.

Fat transfer

Fat transfer for bottom enhancement, also called a Brazilian Butt Lift, is becoming increasing popular and allows you to use your own fat tissue and cells to boost a saggy bottom. Fat is removed from the tummy or thigh area using gentle syringe aspiration, treated and then injected into the bottom cheeks.

Ouch factor: can be a little uncomfortable.

How long will it last? Any fat that has remained after 3 months will last realistically 5 to 10 years.

Reaction

This can also work wonders if your behind isn't too saggy and it'll reduce cellulite, too. See page 208 for a description of the treatment.

Nip tuck know how

Prevention is always the best approach but once gravity and kids have done their worst, you may find that you need surgical help. Some pockets of fat are particularly resistant to all other approaches, and problems such as 'apron tummy' (see below) can't be dealt with in any other way.

THE MOST POPULAR SURGICAL TREATMENTS FOR TUMS AND BUMS

SmartLipo for mummy tummy, midriff bulge and back fat

This is perfect if you have small or medium pockets of fat that won't shift. It's not as aggressive as regular liposuction and you only require a local anaesthetic to numb the area, as well as a little sedation. A tiny laser is inserted just under the skin, melting fat cells, which are then gently sucked out. The laser also stimulates collagen production to tighten the skin. The beauty of SmartLipo is that one or two areas can be treated at the same time. **Downtime:** bruising and swelling for up to two weeks.

BodyTite™ for mummy tummy, droopy bottom, back fat and loose skin

This treatment is particularly good for tightening loose skin as well as reducing surplus fat. A radiofrequency probe is inserted through a tiny incision and it heats and melts fat, which is then sucked out. At the same time a radiofrequency probe heats the skin, causing it to tighten and contract. It requires a local anaesthetic and a little sedation. You'll see results straight away but the full effects kick in between eight and ten weeks later. **Downtime:** you'll be back to normal within a week.

Stem cell-enriched fat transfer for mum bums and stretch marks

This can give droopy bottoms long-lasting curves. The fat will be taken from somewhere you'd rather not have it, such as your hips and thighs, and injected into your buttocks to give them a curvier shape. You'll need a local anaesthetic and sedation.

Downtime: up to a week, and expect bruising and minor swelling. Sitting down is a little sore!

The same technique can be used to replace the fat that's missing under stretch marks. The stem cells enable the fat to graft so it's a permanent solution. You'll only need a local anaesthetic along with sedation and it gives the best results I've ever seen.

Downtime: expect some discomfort but you'll be back to normal in a few days.

Tummy tuck for 'apron tummy'

I always prefer to take the non-surgical route, but there are times when only surgery will do the trick. This is usually the case with 'apron tummy', where there's a lot of loose skin hanging from the abdomen. This can happen if you lose a significant amount of weight and you're left with lots of excess stretched skin. It can also happen after childbirth, especially with twins. A tummy tuck may be your only answer, but ask your surgeon about scarring, as it can be considerable. This has a big ouch factor – the surgeon separates the skin from the wall of the abdomen, then pulls the loose abdominal muscles from the left and right flanks together and sutures them to create a tighter tummy and smaller waist. Excess skin is removed and a new opening is made for the belly button. You have to really want this surgery to go through the procedure!

Downtime: a month before you get back to normal.

Buttock lift for saggy bottom

This can be a really painful op and, again, you have to consider the scarring you'd be left with. If you're only bothered about looking great with your clothes on, this could be for you, but if you're conscious of how you look naked, think very seriously about this surgery. You'll need a general anaesthetic and the procedure takes up to three hours. The surgeon makes an incision, usually along the buttock crease where scars aren't so noticeable, then implants are inserted either under or on top of the muscle.

Downtime: sitting down is very painful for a couple of weeks and bruising and swelling may take several weeks to disappear. It'll take a month to recover.

ten
Show Some Leg

Every year around Easter, my husband utters those ten little words that send shivers down my spine: 'Darling, I think we should book a relaxing beach holiday.' Immediately I'm thrown into a panic thinking about parading around a beach with hardly any clothes on – and showing off my lumpy, bumpy thighs is the most terrifying aspect. Then there are all those other leg issues to contend with: saggy skin, visible veins, wrinkly knees and pale flabby flesh. It doesn't sound so relaxing now, does it?

I don't want every holiday to be a city break, even if they are romantic, and my husband needs a proper rest, so unless I'm content to spend a fortnight in floor-length sarongs, I need a little help in the leg department. And I know I'm not alone. Cellulite in particular is one problem that isn't choosy when it comes to a woman's age, weight or fitness. Even young, super-slim Sienna Miller has admitted to having it, and there are plenty more like her. Snapping gorgeous 20-something starlets with orange-peel thighs is a media obsession, and it's something all but a select few of us can relate to.

Right then, eyes down: what can we do about it?

The problem: cellulite

Cellulite is the stubborn bumpy fat that clings to our thighs and targets women of all ages, shapes and sizes. The effect is often described as cottage cheese or orange peel skin, but I prefer to think of it as like a pocket-sprung mattress. It is actually bulging fat cells enveloped between layers of fibrous tissue. As these fat cells become larger, because of weight gain, hormonal changes or water retention, they squeeze the connective tissues, causing the skin above to pucker and the lymphatic drainage system that removes fluids, toxins and fat naturally is unable to function efficiently.

It's hard to shift because the layer of tissue where cellulite resides doesn't seem to respond to diet or exercise. I've seen many incredibly fit women who have cellulite.

It's more common in women than men because we have more of this type of fibrous tissue. It also appears to be linked to our hormones and develops in those areas where we're genetically programmed to store fat.

The only way to improve the appearance of this hard-to-shift fat is to launch an attack from all sides – diet, exercise, lifestyle and treatments. I hope you're in the mood for a fight!

DIY FIXES

Massage, massage, massage!

This is one of your best options for helping to improve the appearance of dimply thighs. You can use a special anti-cellulite cream, although I don't think it's necessary. These typically contain ingredients such as caffeine to improve micro-circulation and other ingredients to improve skin firmness, but the effects are temporary (see page 129). The action of massage is much more important. Warm some of your chosen cream or oil in your hands then slowly massage your dimply areas, working up your legs using a firm circular motion – try using your knuckles. Working in this way, up towards the heart, will help your lymphatic system to flush out toxins. You'll need to do this religiously at least once a day to see any improvement.

> **TIP!** Try a home-made coffee scrub. Instead of chucking out the used coffee grounds from your machine, massage them into your thighs to help reduce the appearance of bumpy flesh. Many cellulite creams use caffeine as their main active ingredient, so this is just cutting out the middle man! Make sure you stand in the bath or shower to apply your coffee scrub as it can get messy. You could also try adding a little olive oil to the coffee grounds for extra-soft skin.

Brush up!

Dry body brushing helps reduce the appearance of cellulite by improving the texture of your skin. It boosts micro-circulation, helping to clear the build-up of waste and toxins under the skin. Invest in a natural bristle brush – Elemis has a good natural cactus one. Start at your feet and work up towards your thighs, bottom and hips in long sweeping movements. Always brush towards your heart, taking care not to press too hard, and avoid any broken skin. Try to fit in a quick body brush before every shower or bath and see how your skin improves.

Keep moving

Staying active is important. Regular exercise helps your whole body function better, boosting circulation and helping to remove excess toxins from skin tissue. It also helps you lose those extra pounds and improve muscle tone for firmer, smoother-looking thighs. Start by simply building more activity into your week, such as regular walks or activities with the kids. It all adds up.

Junk the junk food

As cellulite is linked to a build-up of toxins, try to eliminate as many of these from your diet as possible – that means limiting alcohol and caffeine, and giving nicotine the boot. You should also ditch processed foods, ready-meals and fast food. Cut down on fatty foods, dairy products and refined carbs, such as white rice and bread and cakes made with white flour. All of these slow down the body's ability to expel the toxins that contribute to cellulite.

Eat more fresh food

To help 'cleanse' your body, include more antioxidant-rich fresh fruit and veg in your diet. The more brightly coloured they are, the more good they'll do you – think carrots, tomatoes, blackberries, blueberries, strawberries, cherries, grapefruit, oranges, mangoes, sweet potato and broccoli. And include more unrefined carbs, such as brown rice and wholegrain bread.

Drink loads of water

I know this is an old chestnut but it really is good for you! Skincare experts like me recommend drinking plenty of water, not because it keeps your skin hydrated – there is no clinical evidence to support that – but because it helps your whole body to function properly. If you get bored with water, try making it more interesting. Add fresh lime, lemon or orange wedges, or a few sprigs of mint. Soda water with a little lime cordial is refreshing. And give herbal teas a whirl. I love fresh mint tea – just add a few sprigs to a cup of warm water or brew it in a teapot.

Take skin-friendly supplements

Take a supplement containing Omega 3, 6, and 9 fatty acids every day. I'm so convinced of their benefits, I've even developed my own supplement called Skin Food. These fatty acids are useful for cellulite because they help the body to metabolise fat and also keep cells healthy and hydrated for healthier-looking skin.

For more on nourishing your skin from within, see pages 58–65.

Fake it

Tanned legs look slimmer and sexier – and somehow cellulite, veins and blemishes don't appear quite so obvious. Fake is the only way to go, though. For more tips on how to achieve a flawless finish with fake tan, see pages 45–8.

> **TIP!** Make the most of your legs (even if you're only exposing them below the knee) by applying some sexy body lotion. Make sure they're super-smooth and hair-free, then slick on a shimmering cream such as Palmer's Cocoa Butter Formula Body Gloss (great for dry skin) or Givenchy Very Irresistible Sensation Body Veil (which is scented, too). Perfect for a glamorous summer evening.

'Fat-melting' pants, anyone?

OK, it's last resort time. You've tried every treatment under the sun and lived like a saint for months and still the dimples won't budge. Could it be time to give a pair of 'miracle pants' a whirl? There are several of these on the market, including Marks & Spencer's Firm Control Waist and Thigh Cincher and Scala Bio-Fir from John Lewis. Woven into the fabric are ingredients such as caffeine and crystals that heat up on contact with skin. The theory is that these pants improve circulation, melting fat, which then drains away naturally. It's recommended you wear them for between six and ten hours a day for a month – which I imagine could get rather uncomfortable and sweaty! You'd need to put a huge amount of heat into the skin to change it and knowing how hard cellulite is to shift, I'm sceptical; but added ingredients such as vitamin E could smooth skin and the firm control fabric will give you a better silhouette under your clothes. Maybe some good body cream and a pair of bog-standard Spanx would do the job just as well, though!

AT THE SALON AND SPA

Have MLD massage

A regular manual lymphatic drainage massage can help give dimply thighs a smoother look. The therapist uses a gentle, rhythmic pumping technique, which stimulates the lymphatic system to remove excess fluid and trapped toxins from cells and body tissue. It's a lovely, relaxing treatment, too.

Elemis also has a good treatment to tackle cellulite called Body Sculpting Cellulite and Colon Therapy, which uses massage techniques to boost lymphatic drainage, alongside a fennel and birch body mask, as well as abdominal massage to stimulate the colon and aid digestion.

Be a water baby

Hydrotherapy – hot tubs and water jets – can help reduce dimpling by improving circulation and aiding good lymph drainage to clear the body of toxins. I can't think of a nicer way of tackling cellulite than relaxing in a warm tub while a jet of water does all the hard work of pummelling my thighs!

Try Endermologie

This French treatment has been popular for several years now. You slip into a body stocking and the therapist massages you with rollers and suction to boost lymphatic drainage and improve skin quality. You'll need between 14 and 28 treatments, administered once or twice a week, and you should start seeing results after six or eight sessions. It's a treatment you need to maintain, so after your initial course I'd recommend monthly top-ups.

... or Ionithermie

This is another treatment from France that's been around for about 30 years, so there must be a few women out there who think it works. These days it's considered old-fashioned, though. After applying a mud or algae mask and essential oils to your bottom and thighs, the therapist hooks you up to electric pads and electrically stimulates the muscles, causing them to tense and relax. This in turn boosts circulation, leaving you with smoother, firmer skin. You'll probably need between six and ten treatments.

> **TIP!** No salon or spa treatment will offer a permanent solution to cellulite, but they can definitely improve the appearance of your thighs, as long as you're also eating well, eliminating the junk from your diet and keeping active. Keep up the hard work or those dimples will just return with a vengeance!

AT THE CLINIC

Reaction

I've mentioned this treatment before in relation to dimply upper arms and I think it is a great option for dimply thighs, too. See page 208 for more information on Reaction.

Ouch factor: there is no downtime and it's not painful, although some women might find it a little uncomfortable.

How long will it last? With yearly top-ups, results will be permanent.

Mesotherapy

This treatment was developed in France in the 1950s and involves micro-injections of pharmaceutical drugs, amino acids and vitamins into the middle layer of the skin to break down fat and clear lymphatic congestion. It needs to be administered by a medical practitioner. I'd suggest between eight and ten treatments initially, with monthly top-ups.

Ouch factor: you might get a pinching sensation with the injections but it's not painful.

How long will it last? If this works for you (it doesn't for everyone), you'll need a top-up yearly.

> **TIP!** It seems every week there's a new weird and wonderful miracle gadget that claims to cure cellulite, from cellulite bikes with infrared beams to cross-trainers that create a vacuum around your lower body. Most of these sessions don't come cheap, so I'd stick with the tried and tested methods, or the ones that don't break the bank. If you don't see benefits after spending a few pounds on a pair of cellulite-busting pants or caffeine tights, it's not such a big deal. But forking out hundreds of pounds for ten sessions on a 'miracle machine' that doesn't achieve what you'd hoped is a whole other ball game.

The problems: inner thigh jiggle and saddlebags

If, like me, you've tried every weird and wonderful diet under the sun but your inner thighs still rub together, let me tell you that we are in the majority. It's a tough area to target and I've even seen gym junkies with this problem, as well as the fat that accumulates on the outside of your thighs – lovingly known as saddlebags. Unfortunately, because of our hormones, women store fat more readily on the lower body, which is why we're more prone to thunder thighs than men. This area is the energy storage for us in anticipation of breast-feeding. But in my experience, once this fat lays itself down, it's very hard to shift. If you're lucky enough not to be a typical English pear shape, congratulate yourself for having such great genes and skip this bit. However, if your thighs could do with a little trimming and toning, read on.

DIY FIXES

Work those thighs!

Build thigh-firming activities into your week. Walking (particularly up hills), climbing stairs and cycling are all good ways to tone up. They'll help burn fat, too. If you're a gym bunny, try the elliptical trainer – it'll strengthen and tone leg muscles without putting stress on the joints.

At home, try these simple moves:

- To firm inner thighs – sit in a sturdy chair with your feet on the floor and place a Swiss ball or a large pillow between your legs. Squeeze the ball or pillow with your thighs and hold for two to three seconds, then release. Do two sets of ten repetitions.

- To firm outer thighs – lie on your side with feet together and toes pointing forwards. Rest your head on the lower outstretched arm and rest the fingers of your upper arm on the floor in front of you for support. Once you're comfortable, raise your upper leg to make an angle of about 40 degrees between your legs, then smoothly lift and lower your leg by a few inches (make sure it doesn't touch your other leg). Aim for ten to twelve lifts, then lie on your other side and repeat.

- To firm the front of your thighs – stand with your upper back against a wall, feet shoulder-width apart, toes pointed slightly outwards. Keeping your back against the wall, inhale and slowly slide down the wall into a squat position, keeping your heels in contact with the floor at all times. Exhale and slowly straighten your legs, returning to the starting position. Aim for eight to ten repetitions.

- To firm the back of your thighs – lie on your back on the floor with your knees bent, then lift your bottom so you're in a 'bridge' position and hold for ten seconds. Slowly lower back down. You should feel a tightening sensation in the backs of your legs. Aim for two sets of ten to twelve repetitions.

- Pick a Power Plate for perfect pins. If you want to tone your legs fast for bikini season, try a Power Plate workout. This vibrating machine has been around for a few years now and is a favourite with A-listers and models because it gets results in weeks rather than months. You hold different positions, such as squats and lunges, on a vibrating platform, which activates muscles to stretch, tone and strengthen.

  Elle 'The Body' Macpherson reported a difference in her legs after using a Power Plate, saying everything was 'so much firmer'. You'll find that most gym groups have Power Plates now.

Pilates

This is great for toning up wobbly thighs. The exercises are designed to develop longer, leaner muscles so your legs will look trim and toned instead of getting bulky, which is what happens with some other workouts. It also improves strength, flexibility and, like yoga, promotes a sense of wellbeing. What's not to love?

Bulge-controlling pants

To minimise jiggle under close-fitting clothes, there are always figure-fixing pants. The ones that will help 'slim' thighs look like cycling shorts. Visit www.figleaves.com, which has a big range of shapewear.

For more on how to de-age your wardrobe and dress for your shape, see pages 101–9.

AT THE SALON

It's a wrap!

Salon body wraps claim to help you lose inches from troublesome spots such as thighs. Sound too good to be true? A study by the University of Westminster proved that the Universal Contour Wrap Classic treatment does produce instant inch loss – and the results were still there 30 days later. A lot of women choose this option before a special event such as a wedding or a beach holiday. First of all, a clay body mask is applied, then you're wrapped in cotton 'bandages' that have been soaked in a warm mineral-rich solution and left to sweat it out under a blanket. I'd recommend at least three treatments for the best results.

AT THE CLINIC

As well as reducing the appearance of cellulite, Reaction (see page 208) can also reduce the circumference of the leg, making it a good first option for tackling thunder thighs. If this doesn't work for you, the easiest and most permanent solution would be to have the fat removed using SmartLipo, which is minimally invasive and not nearly as aggressive as regular liposuction. For more on this, see page 181.

The problem: visible veins

Spider veins – the proper name is telangectasia – are tiny swollen blood vessels just under the skin. They show up on your legs because of the pressure on the vessels caused by sitting or standing for long periods. They can be red, blue or purple and often develop in clusters, like little spider's webs, hence the name.

They're often genetic, but occasionally they can be a result of a trauma, such as deep bruising or surgery. I got mine during pregnancy, which is fairly common, and was told by my doctor that they'd disappear after the birth – but here I am 25 years later and they're still there.

Spider veins are sometimes fed by a deeper-lying varicose vein, so at my clinic we recommend an ultrasound scan before any treatment to check for these, otherwise you may have costly and uncomfortable treatment only to find that more thread veins appear.

DIY FIXES

Get Omega 3 in your diet

Omega 3 fatty acids are thought to stimulate blood circulation. Make sure your diet is rich in salmon, mackerel, sardines and fresh tuna, which

244 • EASY WAYS TO DROP A DECADE

all have high levels of Omega 3. If you're not a fish fan, take a supplement – for extra health benefits, choose one that contains Omega 6 and 9, too.

Be a garlic lover

Not everyone loves the taste of garlic – or the smell that lingers on your breath afterwards. If you don't, try a garlic extract supplement. Allicin, the active ingredient in garlic, is thought to relax blood vessel walls and also make blood less 'sticky', so it's less likely to slow circulation. Try Kwai Garlic supplements.

Enjoy a red wine tipple

At last – an excuse to enjoy that glass of red! Antioxidants called polyphenols, which give red wine its taste and colour, are thought to reduce the build-up of plaque in your arteries to improve blood flow. This isn't the green light for a binge, though – it's all about moderate drinking. The wines with the highest levels of polyphenols are dark reds from Chile and Argentina and the French Malbec and Tannat grape varieties. If you're not a red wine drinker, dark chocolate, walnuts, cranberries and apples also contain polyphenols.

> **TIP!** There are herbal remedies which help with the symptoms of visible veins, including heavy, tired legs. Try A. Vogel Venaforce, which is made from an extract of fresh horse chestnut seeds, or Antistax Red Vine Leaf Extract.

Move around (even when you're sitting)

If you have a spare few minutes during the day, try this exercise to get your blood flowing. Lie on your back and bring one knee up to chest level, clasping your hands behind the knee. Point and flex your foot, then rotate your ankle. Do the same with the other leg. Clasp both hands behind your knees and rotate both ankles at the same time.

Or try this one if you're sitting at work or watching the TV at home. Sit up straight with both feet flat on the floor. Keeping your heels on the floor, tilt your foot off the ground. Lower and repeat 10 times, then do the same with the other foot. Every little helps!

> **TIP!** Mix a couple of drops of lemon balm or lemongrass essential oil with some E45 cream and massage into tired calves and ankles for an exhilarating boost.

Love your winter wardrobe
It's easier to cover unsightly veins in winter. Go for opaque tights rather than sheer hosiery – they're much more on-trend and nothing will show through. Knee-length boots will also do a good job of covering veins on your calves.

Use make-up
You can get camouflage make-up that'll cover up veins. My favourite is Cover FX, a good emergency fix for the summer months.

AT THE CLINIC

Sclerotherapy
The vein is injected with an irritant solution, causing it to collapse and disappear. It's important to wear compression stockings afterwards to help restrict bruising. In my experience it tends to look worse before it gets better. Bruising can last from two weeks to three months depending on

the size of the veins being treated. You'll need between three and six treatments, two to three weeks apart.

Ouch factor: the needle is tiny, but you'll get a stinging sensation.

How long will it last? It can be permanent, although if you're prone to these veins, more could appear.

KTP laser

This works well for leg veins that are too small for sclerotherapy. It is also effective for other vascular blemishes on the leg, such as haemangiomas (cherry red spots) and spider veins. It treats the veins through a series of laser light pulses that are absorbed into the blood, causing the vessels to collapse. Over time (two to four weeks) the treated area returns to the skin's natural colour.

Ouch factor: there is no downtime and the procedure is not painful.

How long will it last? Results are permanent.

Veinwave™

This is a minimally invasive electrical treatment in which an ultra-fine needle is inserted alongside the vein, just under the surface layers of skin. A microwave current is passed through the needle, obliterating the offending vein. The nickel needles are insulated so as not to damage the surrounding tissue. The effect of the treatment is instant – you can literally see the veins disappearing immediately. You may need another treatment after six weeks as some veins can get missed. If you have sensitive skin you can get redness after the treatment, which should disappear in a few days if not hours.

Ouch factor: the sensation is similar to a warm pinprick or minor sting.

How long will it last? The results are excellent, but there's always a chance the spider veins will recur and you may get new ones developing.

Elos eMax

This is one of the few lasers that can treat darker skins. Combined bi-polar radiofrequency and laser energies target and heat unwanted veins, while protecting the surrounding skin. You can see results after a single treatment, but four sessions will produce excellent results. You can have it done in your lunch hour and go back to work afterwards.

Ouch factor: slightly uncomfortable.

How long will it last? The success rate is high, but there's always a chance veins will reappear or new ones will crop up.

Nd Yag Laser

This laser also works well on darker skins. It raises the temperature of spider veins, causing them to collapse and be absorbed by the body. You'll need between four and six treatments, four weeks apart. You can get burnt with this treatment, so make sure you choose an experienced operator. You may get a little redness, swelling and bruising for a few days afterwards.

Ouch factor: yes, this one can hurt! It feels like a strong rubber band being pinged on to the skin as the laser light is pulsed over the vein.

How long will it last? Good results, but a chance you'll get more veins.

Intense pulsed light (IPL)

The IPL heats up the wall of the vein, which then collapses and dissolves. Usually you'll need between three and six treatments a month apart. You can't have the treatment when you have a tan as the light targets pigment, so you could end up with a nasty patch of darker skin. It's definitely a treatment for the winter months. You might get a little redness and bruising afterwards.

Ouch factor: it's uncomfortable, again like an elastic band being pinged on to your skin.

How long will it last? Good success, but as with the other treatments there is a risk that veins will reappear.

The problem: varicose veins

Your veins have tiny one-way valves inside them that open up to let the blood through, then close to stop it from flowing backwards. Sometimes the vein walls stretch and lose their elasticity, which makes the valves weak. When the valves don't function properly, it can cause your blood to leak and flow backwards, collecting in your veins and making them swollen and enlarged. Lovely!

We don't know why some people develop this problem, but women are more likely to be affected by varicose veins than men because female hormones tend to relax the walls of veins. Other factors include being overweight, your genes, pregnancy and jobs where you're standing for long periods, because the blood doesn't flow so easily.

These nasty-looking veins usually appear on the backs of your calves, or on the inside of your leg. Not only does this look ugly, you may also get symptoms such as aching, heavy and uncomfortable legs, swollen feet and ankles, burning or throbbing in your legs, muscle cramps (particularly at night) and dry, itchy, thin skin over the vein.

Here's what can be done about them...

DIY FIXES

Get good habits

Losing weight if you need to will help, and exercise will boost circulation, so keep as active as possible. Raise your legs when you're sitting down and wear compression stockings during the day – these will flatten the veins and help muscles pump blood up to the heart. Maternity compression stockings are available, too. Don't sit on your legs or cross them as this makes it harder for the veins to do their job.

AT THE CLINIC

Endovenous Laser Treatment (EVLT)

EVLT is minimally invasive, requires only a local anaesthetic, and there's less bruising and discomfort after the procedure than traditional surgery. A laser fibre is inserted into the vein through a small cut either just above the knee or in the thigh. It is then slowly withdrawn, damaging the vein's walls and shrinking them closed so blood can no longer flow through it. After treatment, an elastic stocking bandage is applied and you can walk around within an hour. You can go home the same day, too.

For large veins, you may need surgery (see page 256).

The problem: wrinkly, saggy knees

Knee wrinkles are caused by dehydrated skin, sun damage, loss of skin elasticity, huge weight loss and, of course, advancing years. The skin on your knees gets drier than many other areas of the body because there are fewer oil glands, so it needs a little extra attention.

When my mum was a dancer, some of the older ladies wore flesh-coloured nylons under their fishnets to banish any sign of saggy knees. I'm not sure this would be a good look close up – stick to the opaques, which will keep everything nicely covered and look good, too.

DIY FIXES

Scrub up and nourish

Start by improving the condition of the skin on and around your knees. Use a body brush to improve micro-circulation and bring nutrients to the skin, improving its tone and texture. Use an exfoliator regularly to slough away the build-up of dead skin cells and get rid of flakiness. My favourite is Jan Marini Bioglycolic® Resurfacing Body Scrub.

Massage in an extra-hydrating body cream daily or, better still, treat the area to some of your anti-ageing face cream. The odd face mask is a good quick fix when your knees are going to be on display. Remember to feed your skin from the inside, too, with a good multivitamin and an Omega 3, 6 and 9 supplement.

> **TIP!** For an emergency fix, try some Clarins Beauty Flash Balm on crêpey knees before a night out. It'll temporarily smooth and boost the look of your skin.

AT THE CLINIC

Fraxel Repair laser

This laser is great for a no-knife face-lift (see page 161) and it has the same effect on your knees – tightening the skin by about 30% and stimulating new collagen. There's a bit of downtime with two weeks of redness and peeling, but the results are really good. You'll notice a slight improvement after a week and the quality of your skin will keep on improving over six months.

Ouch factor: this laser hurts!

How long will it last? Up to five years.

Thermage

This radiofrequency treatment puts a lot of heat into your skin to encourage collagen production. It might take a few months before you start seeing an improvement so you have to be patient. It can achieve good

A word about cankles!

Cankles, for those of you who don't know, means calves and ankles that run into each other to give you thick ankles. No diet is going to make a difference to these – you've probably inherited them from your mum or granny. If they really bother you, the only way to change them is by having the fat gently sucked out with SmartLipo – see page 184.

results, though, and your skin will continue to improve over six months. It works best on younger skins, so not for the over-65s.

Ouch factor: yes, it gets quite hot! But there's no downtime.

How long will it last? Several years.

The problem: 'old lady feet'

Our feet get a hard time of it. We spend all day walking on them, we squeeze them into unsuitable shoes with pointy toes and killer heels, we completely ignore them in winter beneath socks and tights, then in summer we run around barefoot. I admit it can be a bit of a chore to look after your feet, particularly when they're not on show most of the time. But come summer, when the shops are full of gorgeous strappy sandals, you'll wish you'd taken better care of them. When I think of 'old lady feet', I think of calluses, hard skin, discoloured nails that haven't seen a lick of polish, never mind a file, in a long time and, of course, bunions. Urrgh! No amount of Jimmy Choos or Manolo Blahniks will dress up that little lot.

Here's how to get sexier feet.

DIY FIXES

Foot files

The first step to sweeter feet is to get rid of all that nasty rough, hard skin. Every time you have a bath or shower, use a foot file to slough off any hard skin that's formed on your heels, the balls of your feet or the big toes. I think foot files are easier to use than a pumice stone. If you can, go for a stainless steel one, which will be pricier than a regular foot file, but it's much more effective and lasts a long time. SpaceNK has a good one. If you use your foot file regularly, it'll stop the build-up of hard skin so you can avoid a trip to the chiropodist to have it removed professionally.

Pedi cream

My secret weapon against hard skin is Mavala Conditioning Moisturiser For Feet. Beauty editors are always raving about the benefits of this product and I couldn't agree more. It contains marine collagen to prevent dry skin and leaves feet ultra soft. For an added treat, slather on an extra helping, put on a pair of thick socks and wear overnight.

Enjoy a DIY foot spa and pedicure

No time or money for a professional pedicure? Then treat your feet to a little at-home pampering. Here's how.

Step 1: soak your feet in a bath of warm water with Epsom salts and a few drops of your favourite essential oil for about 10 minutes. A large glass bowl or a washing-up basin are perfect for this. Proper foot spas with bubbling water are a nice luxury, but I think they're a pain to store when you're not using them.

Step 2: after patting your feet dry, it's time to exfoliate. There are plenty of foot scrubs to choose from – try The Body Shop Peppermint Soothing Foot Scrub or make your own using olive oil mixed with either sugar or sea salt. Rub the exfoliator all over your feet, paying special attention to dry, hard skin, then take it about halfway up your calves. Rinse off in the foot bath and gently pat dry.

Step 3: smooth on loads of nourishing foot cream and massage it in well, using your thumbs in a firm press-release motion from the bottom of your arch to the base of your toes. Afterwards wipe nails with a tissue to get rid of any excess cream in preparation for polish.

Step 4: now it's time to get nicer nails. Start by trimming them with nail scissors or clippers (they should be short and square). It's OK to file them straight across to get rid of rough edges and make them even, but don't file away the corners as this can lead to an ingrown nail. Next, use a nail buffer to smooth ridges and get rid of any superficial discolouration. Apply a base coat to avoid the polish staining your nails and provide a smoother surface for it to adhere to. Now apply two coats of polish and finish with a topcoat to seal the colour and help prevent chips and fading. Your polish should last between two and three weeks. For longer-lasting shine and colour, apply a fresh layer of topcoat once every two or three days.

Three of my favourite foot creams

- Avon Footworks Therapeutic Cracked Heel Relief Cream – as with many Avon products, this one is a bargain and great for softening calluses and dry, cracked skin. It fights infection, too.
- Neutrogena Norwegian Formula 24 Hour Moisturisation Foot Cream – this contains glycerine and vitamin E to lock in moisture. A good high street choice.
- NeoStrata Foot Gel Plus – this extra-strength formula includes 15% glycolic acid – my favourite ingredient! It exfoliates, smooths and softens all in one go – what's not to love?

The problem: bunions

There's nothing that'll age your feet more than a pair of whopping great bunions. Just ask Victoria Beckham, who famously stepped out of her trademark seven-inch heels into some rather less glamorous flip-flops, revealing monster bunions. Ouch! The official name for a bunion is hallux valgus – even that sounds horrible – and it develops when the big toe becomes angled in towards your other toes. This forces the bone at the base of the big toe to stick out at the side. Irritation of the soft tissue can cause further swelling and pain.

Bunions can be a hereditary problem but, more often than not, they're caused by ill-fitting shoes, which is why so many younger women now suffer from them. Killer courts with pointy fronts that force your toes into a cramped space are the worst offenders. Shoes like these can even cause a bunion on your little toe, which is known quite sweetly as a bunionette!

When it comes to treating them, you can try bunion pads to relieve pressure, special insoles and painkillers. Choosing a shoe with a mid-heel and a more rounded toe with more wiggle room will also help. If they become very swollen and painful, your only answer is surgery to remove the bunion and realign the bones. Afterwards walking can be difficult for

TIP! Give your feet a break! If you're out for the night in towering stilettos, keep a pair of ballet flats in your bag for the journey home. Try Rollasole, a clever, bargain ballet pump that roles up small enough to fit into a clutch bag. Bloch Roll Up Ballet Flats are also good. And don't walk for any distance in your heels. Put them in a bag and pop on some trainers instead. Your feet will thank you for it!

a few weeks and you'll need to wear wide-fitting, low-heeled shoes for around six months.

Nip tuck know how

You know what I'm going to say – treat surgery as the last resort. Always try the non-surgical alternatives first. And if you opt for an operation, do your research thoroughly. Here's my lowdown on what's available.

THE MOST POPULAR SURGICAL TREATMENTS FOR LEGS AND FEET

SmartLipo for dimply, wobbly thighs

This minimally invasive treatment can remove excess fat and smooth the skin. A fibre optic laser is inserted through tiny incisions to melt the fat, which is gently sucked out through a cannula. The fibre is then reinserted under the skin to tighten it. You'll need a local anaesthetic and a little sedation. Some results will be visible immediately but you'll need to wait for the swelling to go down to see the full effect.

Downtime: you'll have bruising and swelling for up to two weeks.

Liquid Lipo or LipoSoft

This is a newer treatment and not one of my favourites. It involves having water injected into the fatty area to help push nerves and blood vessels out of the path of the cannula. It minimises the amount of damage to the tissue and ultimately reduces recovery time by limiting bruising and swelling. It also makes the treatment more comfortable.

Downtime: any pain can be controlled with painkillers, although you may still feel stiff and sore for a few days and it always takes a little time to recover from a general anaesthetic.

BodyTite™ for wrinkly, saggy knees

With this treatment, a probe is inserted under the skin while another rests on the skin surface. Radiofrequency energy is transmitted between the probes, causing the breakdown of fat cells, which are sucked out. Heating the skin causes it to shrink, tighten and thicken. You'll need a local anaesthetic and sedation.

Downtime: you'll be out of action for a week but the results are excellent and your skin will keep improving over the next six months as more collagen is produced. It's a great treatment for loose skin.

Thigh lift for loose skin on knees and thighs

Ouch! This is real surgery and should only be considered if you have a lot of loose skin hanging around your knees as the result of dramatic weight loss. An incision is made in your groin, then excess skin is cut away and the thigh is literally pulled up and stitched back. Scarring is permanent, but can be hidden in the crease of the thigh. It'll be very sore for up to six weeks and expect considerable bruising and swelling. The results are good but, unlike BodyTite™, the quality of your skin won't be improved and it can become loose again over the next 18 months.

Downtime: you won't be able to drive or exercise for between four and six weeks.

Surgery for varicose veins

Large varicose veins sometimes have to be removed surgically, which involves a general anaesthetic, but you can usually go home the same day. The technique is called ligation and stripping; this means tying off and then removing the varicose vein in the leg. Two small cuts are made, one in your groin at the top of the varicose vein, the other further down your leg, around the knee or ankle. The top part of your vein is tied and sealed, then a thin wire is inserted through the vein and pulled gently out of the cut at the other end. There's a lot of bleeding and bruising as the vein is literally ripped out, but the results are good.

Downtime: you'll have bruising and swelling, and must wear a compression stocking for a week. You'll be able to return to work within three weeks.

Cellulaze

Cellulaze is a new laser treatment for cellulite, and the first and only one that targets the actual structural problems underneath the skin. The tip of the laser is shaped like a pen and is inserted just below the skin to melt

Foot surgery

The number of cosmetic procedures performed on feet has doubled in the last year. From toe shortening or lengthening to a 'pinky tuck' or 'Loub job', women are now opting to undergo this type of surgery simply because their feet look ugly or won't fit into their trendy shoes. But be warned: the risks associated with cosmetic foot surgery far outweigh the benefits. For instance, toe-shortening is extremely painful as it involves the surgeon sawing through bone. The pinky tuck, during which thickened skin on the small toe is removed while the bone is shaved or straightened, is just as painful. The Loub job, nicknamed after shoe designer Christian Louboutin, involves injecting a dermal filler into the toes, heels and balls of the feet in order to cushion them when wearing heels – this costs around £500 and is not permanent. Recovery from foot surgery can take months and carries the risks of nerve injury and prolonged swelling as it is very hard for feet to drain fluid. The foot is a complicated structure and it is not possible to alter one part of it without affecting another. Give this type of surgery a wide berth unless you really have painful or deformed feet.

away superficial fat and increase collagen production. Results are seen after one treatment, but improvements continue to show for up to a year afterwards as new collagen is formed.

Ouch factor: the procedure can be slightly uncomfortable so is performed under local anaesthetic.

How long will it last? Results are permanent.

Conclusion

So, ladies, here we are at the end of the book. I've loved sharing all my anti-ageing secrets and I hope they've inspired you to believe it's possible for each and every one of you to look younger for longer.

I especially hope you feel empowered to take all those DIY fixes and make them work for you, because there is so much you can do yourself to hold back the years. Whether it's good skincare habits, diet and lifestyle tweaks, a make-up bag makeover, a wardrobe revamp or a sexy new haircut – all of them can give your confidence an amazing boost. And there's nothing more attractive and vital than a woman who is happy in her own skin and knows she looks good.

If you feel you're ready for a little extra cosmetic help – whether that's Botox or a bottom lift – you now know what to expect from these procedures and how to go about choosing one that's right for you.

The fact is, we live longer these days, so it's completely natural to want to prolong our looks, health and vitality for as long as we can. But, as I've said before, for me, looking younger for longer is not about vanity or desperately trying to recreate the way we looked in our 20s. It's about continuing to live our lives to the full despite those advancing years, looking and feeling the absolute best that we can.

And I think we all deserve it.

Your Anti-ageing Glossary

The language that's used to describe anti-ageing treatments, ingredients and products can be utterly mystifying. Here's my easy jargon-busting guide to the beauty business.

A is for...

AHAs (alpha hydroxy acids) Natural acids found in fruit and milk that can help reduce fine lines, smooth skin, and unblock pores. AHAs gently exfoliate by breaking down the 'glue-like' substance that holds dead skin cells together. Those most commonly used in skin cream and treatments include citric acid, glycolic acid and lactic acid.

Airgent™ A high-speed jet that introduces hyaluronic acid (qv) into the skin to generate collagen production, which will thicken and tighten skin.

Antioxidants These natural nutrients help the body fight against ageing free radicals. You can get the benefit of antioxidants by including them in your diet and your skincare products. Key antioxidants include flavonoids, alpha lipoic acid, Coenzyme Q10 (qv) and vitamins A, C and E.

Argeriline (also known as Argireline or acetyl hexapeptide-3) A synthetic peptide that can relax facial muscles without paralysing them, and so soften wrinkles. It's often touted by beauty companies as a non-invasive alternative to Botox (qv), as it works in a similar but less dramatic way. It's used in anti-ageing creams and must be applied daily to maintain results.

Azzalure® The brand name of a botulinum toxin similar to Botox (qv). It's injected in the same way to smooth facial wrinkles by relaxing muscles.

B is for...

BHA (beta hydroxy acid) A group of naturally occurring acids, these are often used to exfoliate dead skin cells and sebum, and can also be anti-inflammatory and antibacterial. Salicylic acid is the best known BHA, commonly used in acne treatments.

Bio Gel therapy Uses your own growth factors (taken from your blood) and injects them into skin to repair acne scars and reduce wrinkles.

Blepharoplasty Popular surgery to improve the appearance of eye bags and crow's feet, by removing excess skin and fat from around the eyes. Performed under general anaesthetic.

BodyTite™ A method of body reshaping, which safely melts and removes fat and simultaneously tightens loose skin.

Botox The brand name for botulinum toxin, which blocks the chemical responsible for telling muscles to contract. Injecting it into facial muscles relaxes them, erasing wrinkles for up to six months.

Brachioplasty Commonly known as an arm lift, this surgery is used to reduce bingo wings and tighten skin on the upper arms, by removing excess fat and skin under general anaesthetic.

Breast implants Artificial implants used to enlarge and shape the breasts.

Breast reduction A surgical operation to reduce the size and weight of the breasts. Fat, glandular tissue and skin is removed, then breasts are reshaped and repositioned.

C is for...

Cellulite Stubborn, lumpy fat that gives a dimpled or uneven appearance to skin and is commonly found around the thighs, bottom and upper arms.

Ceramides Naturally-occurring oils, often added to anti-ageing products because they help strengthen the skin's protective barrier, so it can retain moisture and stay smooth and soft.

Chemical peels A treatment to freshen skin, remove pigmentation and reduce fine lines and scarring. A naturally occurring acid such as glycolic (from sugar cane), salicylic (from willow bark) or kojic (from mushrooms) is applied to the face, causing the surface layers of skin to peel off, revealing a more youthful complexion. There are different strengths of peel – from mild to deep – depending on the condition of your skin.

Cinderella Lips In this treatment, lips are enhanced using a liquid injection that only lasts a few days, so you can see if you like the effect before opting for anything more long-term.

CO_2 laser resurfacing Carbon dioxide lasers use very short pulses of light energy or continuous light beams to remove thin layers of skin with great precision. These are used to treat wrinkles, acne, skin lumps and bumps and scars.

Coenzyme Q10 (CoQ10) A nutrient found naturally in the body, which helps cells function properly and fight ageing. As we age, our body produces less of it, slowing down the skin's collagen and elastin production and causing wrinkles. Supplements or creams containing this ingredient may help boost skin regeneration and fight ageing.

Collagen Skin is made mainly of the protein collagen, which works with elastin to give it a youthful, plump appearance. Sun damage and ageing cause collagen in the skin to deteriorate. The goal of most skin rejuvenation treatments is to stimulate new collagen using lasers or other techniques.

Cosmeceutical A skin product that falls between a drug and a cosmetic because it has higher concentrations of active ingredients than regular beauty products, and has a stronger effect on skin.

Cosmetic acupuncture In this treatment, based on the principles of Oriental medicine, hair-thin needles are inserted into particular areas of the face, ears, neck, hands, trunk and legs along channels or meridians of energy called *qi*. It can help to lift specific areas of the face, improve skin tone, boost blood flow, soften lines and reduce puffiness and eye bags.

D is for...

Dermal fillers A non-surgical treatment in which an ingredient, commonly hyaluronic acid (qv), is injected into the skin to plump it and smooth out lines. Dermal fillers can also be used to fill out the lips, plump out hollow cheeks, reshape the chin or nose tip, or fill acne scars. Results usually last six to eight months.

Dysport® An injectable treatment for wrinkles, made from the same type of neurotoxin, botulinum toxin type A, as Botox (qv).

E is for...

Elastin A stretchy substance in the skin that works with collagen to give skin its youthful flexibility, allowing it to snap back after it is stretched. Natural ageing and sun damage cause the elastin in your skin to deteriorate. Laser treatments can help stimulate new elastin production.

Elos eMax One of the few lasers that can be used on darker skins, this is good for hair reduction and treating spider veins.

Endermologie The most well-known salon treatment to reduce cellulite, which involves massaging the area with small rollers and stimulating skin with suction. Treatments must be kept up to maintain results.

Essential fatty acids (EFAs) EFAs such as Omega 3 and 6 are vital nutrients for maintaining healthy skin, nails and hair. Eating foods rich in EFAs, such as oily fish, nuts and seeds, or taking supplements will ensure a plentiful supply.

Essential oils Concentrated oils from plants, used in products for their fragrance and treatment properties. For example, rose oil benefits mature and sensitive skin, while tea tree oil is anti-bacterial and can fight acne.

EVLT (endovenous laser treatment) This treats varicose veins without the need to remove them, by using a very narrow optical fibre. The treatment can be done under local anaesthetic.

F is for...

Fat transfer injection As it sounds, this is a procedure whereby excess fat can be removed from one part of the body, where it is not wanted, and injected into another part of the body, to plump it up.

Fraxel Repair A laser used to 'resurface' the skin (see Laser resurfacing, below).

Free radicals Highly reactive particles, which are produced both naturally by the body as we age and by outside influences such as cigarette smoke, sun exposure and stress. Free radicals attack and damage cells and break down collagen in the skin, leading to wrinkles and ageing.

G *is for...*

Glycolic acid The smallest alpha hydroxy acid (AHA, qv). It is used in anti-ageing and acne skincare products to remove dead skin build-up and clear blocked pores.

H *is for...*

Humectants Moisturising ingredients, most commonly glycerine, ceramides or lecithin, which are used in face creams as they attract and hold water in the skin.

Hyaluronic acid Found naturally in young skin, hyaluronic acid retains water like a sponge and helps keeps skin moisturised and plump, but over time our skin produces less, causing sagging and loss of tone. It can be added to skin creams to fight lines or injected as a temporary filler to restore plumpness.

Hydroquinone A skin lightening agent used topically to remove dark patches from hyper-pigmented areas of skin. Only available on prescription.

Hydrotherapy Water therapy using jets of hot and cold water as well as hot tubs to stimulate circulation and improve skin tone.

Hyperpigmentation The darkening of a patch of skin caused by increased melanin production.

Hypoallergenic A product labelled hypoallergenic should have been tested and found to be unlikely to cause an allergic reaction or skin irritation.

I *is for...*

Infrared light therapy Originally used in hospitals to heal wounds, this kind of light therapy can have a rejuvenating effect on age-damaged skin.

The infrared light stimulates the production of collagen to help speed up the skin's healing process.

Injectables This term refers to dermal-filler and muscle-relaxing injections.

Intense pulsed light (also known as IPL or photo rejuvenation) Used for hair removal, reducing thread veins, to treat acne and to fight wrinkles, this recently developed therapy uses intense bursts of red or blue light to penetrate the skin's deeper layer and stimulate healing.

Invisible bra A surgical breast-lifting procedure in which a mesh cone a bit like a bra cup is placed underneath the skin to hold the breast in place.

Ionithermie A treatment that uses rhythmic electrical pulses through the tissue to improve the appearance of cellulite and smooth skin texture.

J is for...

Jessner peel A medium-to-strong chemical peel that takes off the top layer of dead skin to treat acne or reduce the appearance of wrinkles and sun damage.

K is for...

Keloid scars An abnormal kind of scar that can form when skin is damaged. Typified by a raised overgrowth of scar tissue, often thick, red, rubbery and larger than the original wound. Darker skins are more prone and the problem may run in families. Cosmetic surgery is best avoided by people prone to keloid scars.

L is for...

Lanolin A fatty substance obtained from wool that has superb moisturising qualities and is used in soaps, cosmetics, and ointments. Can cause a reaction in sensitive skins.

Laser bra lift In this type of breast-lift surgery, a piece of your own skin is used as a strap to lift and support the breast internally.

Laser hair removal A laser delivers a pulsed beam, which is absorbed by the pigment in the hair follicle. As the light converts into heat, it damages the hair follicle and destroys its ability to regrow, resulting in permanent hair reduction.

Laserlipolysis In this treatment, a laser heats unwanted fat deposits so that they melt and can be gently aspirated.

Laser resurfacing In this treatment a laser is used to pierce thousands of tiny holes in your skin, removing the top layers, reducing wrinkles, sun damage and tightening the skin by up to 30%. It also stimulates collagen production to thicken the skin and give it a more youthful appearance.

Laser skin lift There is no cutting, scarring, or anaesthetic with this procedure. Using a laser, the outer layers of the skin are resurfaced and tightened, resulting in fewer fine lines and wrinkles, and lifted skin.

Lightening agents These are used to treat hyperpigmentation (qv).

Lipids Oily substances found naturally in the skin that keep it soft, supple and protected. Examples include sebum and ceramides. They can also be added to beauty products to help increase the skin's moisture content.

Liposomes A clever new ingredient in anti-ageing skincare, liposomes are tiny bubbles made out of the same material as a skin cell membrane and with the ability to penetrate deep into the skin. The bubbles are filled with active ingredients, which are then delivered down to the deepest layers of the skin where they can be most effective.

Liposuction The surgical removal of fat deposits, through a small suction tube inserted under the skin. Liposuction is most commonly used on the thighs or midriff. See SmartLipo, below, for a less aggressive form of fat removal.

Liquid Lipo/LipoSoft A water jet containing local anaesthetic is sprayed out of a cannula at high pressure, breaking up fat cells, which can then be sucked out of the treatment zone. Ouch!

Lumixyl™ A skin-brightening cream used topically to fade skin pigmentation.

Lymphatic system A vital part of the body's natural defence system, which removes toxins and waste products from tissue and cells.

Lypastyle A low-frequency ultrasound treatment, which affects the elasticity of cell membranes causing them to release stored fat into surrounding tissue. The body then disposes of the fat naturally.

M is for...

Macrolane™ A thick dermal filler that is made of hyaluronic acid (qv). It is injected into the breasts or bottom to give fullness.

Manual lymphatic drainage (MLD) A relaxing form of massage that gently stimulates the lymphatic system, encouraging the removal of toxins and fluid build-up. It can reduce puffy eyes and speed healing after cosmetic surgery.

Mesotherapy A therapy that injects tiny amounts of ingredients such as vitamins, amino acids and hyaluronic acid (qv) just millimetres under the skin. This can fight ageing by restoring vital skin nutrients, and it's also used to treat cellulite.

Microdermabrasion A 'sanding down' of the top layer of dead skin using a fine particle spray of either aluminium crystals or salt. It's used in salon facials for a deep exfoliation and to smooth fine lines, revealing younger, more radiant skin underneath.

Micro-needling A drum-shaped instrument covered in tiny needles is rolled over the skin. The needles penetrate the upper layers, stimulating collagen formation and helping anti-ageing skin products to be absorbed more effectively.

Microtox A procedure in which very small amounts of Botox (qv) are injected superficially all over the face to erase wrinkles. It can be used on the forehead, cheeks and sides of the face, around eyes and on the neck.

Mineral oil A by-product of petroleum, this is used in lots of lotions, but clogs pores, causing spots to form.

N is for...

Nanospheres One of the very newest skincare innovations. When used in skin creams, these microscopic particles contain active ingredients, such as antioxidants, and have the ability to penetrate the skin at its deepest level, where they gradually deliver the ingredient for maximum effectiveness.

Nd Yag Laser A type of laser that works well on darker skins. It has a range of cosmetic uses, including the treatment of spider veins.

Niacinamide (also called vitamin B3 or niacin) Topical application of niacinamide has been shown to increase moisture in skin and help with discolouration. It is also a vasodilator, meaning it widens the blood vessels to stimulate circulation, which can counteract dull-looking skin.

Non-comedogenic A product with this label has been tested to ensure it won't block the pores in your skin and trigger spot breakouts.

Novabel® One of the newer dermal fillers used to plump up sagging skin, soften lines and reshape facial features.

O is for...

Omega fatty acids Omega 3 and 6 are essential fatty acids (qv), which means they are essential for good health, but our bodies cannot manufacture them so we must get them from our diet. Omega 9 is a fatty acid that's manufactured by our bodies, so we won't keel over if we don't get it from our diet. All are needed for normal tissue function in the body, including healthy skin, hair and nails.

Oxygen facials A non-surgical treatment involving a high-pressure blast of oxygen that helps feeds serums packed with vitamins, minerals and collagen into your skin. The facial boosts oxygen levels in the skin, resulting in better circulation and skin cell regeneration, which leaves the skin glowing.

P is for...

Panthenol (pro-vitamin B5) A penetrating moisturising ingredient that smoothes skin, strengthens nails and hydrates the hair shaft to make it appear thicker and shinier and reduce split ends.

Parabens Preservatives used in skincare that can cause irritation.

Peel A treatment that strips off the top layer of dead skin cells to reveal fresher skin underneath.

Peptides (can include pentapeptides and hexapeptides) Peptides are chains of amino acids that are present naturally in the body. Synthetic versions are added to skincare products to stimulate collagen, plump up lines and relax wrinkles.

pH level This is a term used to measure the acidity or alkalinity of your skin. Normal skin's pH is between 4.5 and 6.5. Skincare products tend to be more gentle if they have a similar pH level to skin.

Photo-ageing Premature breakdown of skin cells caused by damage from the sun's UVA and UVB rays, and resulting in lines, wrinkles and age spots.

Polyphenols Antioxidants that have anti-inflammatory benefits and can help rejuvenate damaged skin. Anti-ageing skincare products often contain polyphenols sourced from green tea, olive oil and grape seeds.

PRP (platelet-rich plasma) Derived from our blood, this has a high concentration of growth factors that are essential for regeneration and repair of skin. See also Bio Gel therapy.

R is for...

Radiofrequency remodelling A heat treatment to shrink scars and tighten skin. It can also be used to treat bingo wings by tightening the skin and reducing fat.

Radiage A non-invasive wrinkle treatment that uses radiofrequency to tighten and tone skin.

Red light When used as a facial treatment, certain frequencies of red light can stimulate new cell growth to improve skin elasticity and diminish wrinkles, sun damage and broken capillaries.

Restylane® The brand name for a popular hyaluronic acid dermal filler that is injected into the face to fill wrinkles and plump lips.

Resveratrol One of the most potent anti-ageing antioxidants in skin cream, which may slow down the ageing process, fight lines and protect skin collagen.

Retin-A This is a vitamin A derivative that stimulates skin turnover and is used as a topical wrinkle or acne treatment. It is also used as an exfoliant pre-treatment in chemical peels. It is only available on prescription.

Retinoids and retinol Vitamin A derivatives that deeply penetrate the skin to increase cell turnover and strengthen and replenish collagen and elastin. They exfoliate, unclog pores, plump up skin and minimise the appearance of wrinkles, scars and age spots. But they also make the skin more sensitive to sunlight.

Roaccutane A strong synthetic form of vitamin A used to treat acne by dramatically reducing the amount of oil the skin produces.

S is for...

Salicylic acid Originally derived from the bark of the willow tree, it is a beta hydroxy acid that is used in acne treatments.

Sclerotherapy An injected saline- or alcohol-based treatment for spider veins.

Sculptra® An injectable volumising treatment that stimulates your own collagen and is used to fill out tear troughs, hollow cheeks, nose to mouth lines and marionette lines.

Semi-permanent make-up A process in which colour is 'tattooed' into the top layer of the skin, usually used to line the eyes or lips. It lasts for several years, breaking down and fading with time.

Silicone A skincare ingredient with water-repellent properties that protects the skin's moisture levels. Also used to make the most popular kind of breast implants (qv).

SmartLipo A laser-assisted form of liposuction that's used to remove small or medium-sized pockets of fat from various areas of the body.

Smartxide A CO_2 laser (qv) that shrinks skin and stimulates collagen production. It's excellent for skin rejuvenation and for treating acne.

Sodium lauryl sulfate A chemical used to produce lather in cleansers and shampoos, which can cause skin irritation.

SPF (sun protection factor) The level of sun protection a skin cream offers. The higher the level, the longer you can stay in the sun without burning. Factor 15 is considered the minimum for preventing premature ageing.

Stem cell-enriched fat transfer Fat is taken from places you don't want it (such as hips and thighs), processed with your own stem cells, then injected into hands, face, breasts and even your bottom to give volume or plump out lines. The stem cells help the fat 'graft' so it lasts longer.

T is for...

Thermage An anti-ageing treatment that uses a radiofrequency machine to heat the collagen fibres in the skin and thus increase collagen production. This helps tighten skin and softens wrinkles.

Tocopherol A form of vitamin E that, when added to skincare, can help prevent free radical damage, strengthen capillary walls and fight wrinkles.

Trichloroacetic acid (TCA) Used in chemical peels. It's excellent for 'spot' peeling of specific areas, such as the face, neck and hands, removing the top layer of skin to reveal the fresher, smoother skin underneath.

U is for...

UVA Sunlight is composed of UVA and UVB light. UVA is the type of ultraviolet light that can penetrate deep into the skin and can cause wrinkling (photo-ageing), sagging, dry skin and even skin cancer. Prolonged exposure to UVA cracks and shrinks collagen and elastin, causing skin to sag.

UVB The type of ultraviolet light that damages the top layer on the skin. UVB rays stimulate the production of melanin, which makes your skin become tanned – a sign of damage. It also causes sunburn, age spots and is linked to skin cancer.

V is for…

VeinWave™ A non-invasive treatment to treat visible veins.

Vistabel® Another trade name for botulinum toxin, the treatment that is injected into facial muscles to relax wrinkles.

Vitamin A An antioxidant which, when added to skin products, can aid skin renewal and help reverse the signs of photo-ageing.

Vitamin B Vitamins B3 (niacin) and B5 (pantothenic acid) are popular additions to skin products because they help trap moisture.

Vitamin C (also known as L-ascorbic acid) An antioxidant that is essential for the formation of collagen. When applied to your skin, vitamin C can decrease the effects of sun exposure, aid in the production of collagen, fight wrinkle-causing free radicals, and slow the production of age spots.

Vitamin K Strengthens the capillary walls. It can be effective in skincare products for people with rosacea.

Z is for…

Zinc oxide
A proven natural UV blocker that forms the basis of many sunscreens. Good for sensitive skins.

Stockists

For Harley Street skin products, visit our website
www.harleystreetskincare.co.uk

For all other products recommended in this book, if you can't find them
in your local chemist or department store, use the websites listed below
to find the stockists nearest to you, or to order online.

Antistax www.antistax.co.uk
Avene www.avene.co.uk
A.Vogel Venaforce www.avogel.co.uk
Avon www.avon.uk.com
Barefoot Botanicals www.barefoot-botanicals.com
Beauty Lab www.beautylab.co.uk
Benefit www.benefitcosmetics.co.uk
Bio-Oil available from Boots
Bloch Roll Up Ballet Flats www.endless.com
B. Kamins www.salonskincare.co.uk
Bobbi Brown www.bobbibrown.co.uk
Body Shop www.thebodyshop.co.uk
Boots www.boots.com
Bourjois available from Boots

BPC www.mineralearth.co.uk or www.ilovebeautyproducts.com

Brush Up www.mineralearth.co.uk

Burt's Bees www.burtsbees.co.uk

Caudalie www.caudalie.com/uk

Cetaphil www.cetaphil.co.uk

Chantecaille www.spacenk.co.uk

Clairol www.clairol.co.uk

Clarins available from all large department stores

Clinique www.clinique.co.uk

Compression stockings www.compressionstockings.co.uk

Cosmedicine www.beautybay.com

Cover FX www.coverfx.com

Dermajuv www.treatyourskin.co.uk

Dermalogica www.dermalogica.com/uk

Dermaroller www.genuinedermaroller.co.uk

Dr Brandt Pores No More www.spacenk.co.uk

Dr Hauschka www.drhauschka.co.uk

Dr Organics available from Holland & Barrett

Elemis www.timetospa.co.uk and www.elemis.com

Elizabeth Arden www.elizabetharden.co.uk

Essential oils www.essentialoilsonline.co.uk

Estée Lauder available from all large department stores

Eylure www.eylure.com

Facial-Flex www.rosemaryconley.com

Fake Bake www.fakebake.co.uk

Freeze 24-7 www.freeze247.com

Frownies www.frownies.co.uk

Gatineau Gatineau.SalonSkincare.co.uk

Givenchy www.givenchy.com

GloMinerals www.glomineralsmakeup.com

HSS www.harleystreetskincare.co.uk

Huit, Just A Kiss Padded Shorty www.figleaves.com

Ilift www.iliftuk.com

Iman cosmetics www.imancosmetics.com

Jan Marini www.ilovebeautyproducts.com

Jurlique www.jurlique.co.uk

Kettlebell www.kettlebells.co.uk

Kwai Garlic supplements available from health stores

La Decollette bras www.decollette.eu

Laura Mercier www.spacenk.co.uk

Liz Earle www.lizearle.com

Lumixyl www.lumixyl.com

Mac www.maccosmetics.co.uk

Mama Mio www.mamamio.com

Mavala www.mavala.co.uk

Max Factor www.maxfactor.co.uk

Maxi Lip Plump www.lovethymakeup

Maybelline www.maybelline.co.uk

MD Formulations www.salonskincare.co.uk

Medik8 www.medik8.co.uk

Mineral Earth www.mineralearth.co.uk

Miraclesuit swimwear www.lingeriebrands.co.uk

Nair www.naircare.co.uk

Natural Skin Solutions www.shopwiki.co.uk

NeoStrata www.ilovebeautyproducts.com

Neutrogena available from Boots, most pharmacies

Not Your Daughter's Jeans www.nydj.com

Olay available from Boots, most pharmacies

Opi www.nailsandthings.co.uk

The Organic Pharmacy www.theorganicpharmacy.com

Palmer's www.superdrug.com

Prescriptives www.prescriptives.co.uk

Rejuve www.rejuve-mask.co.uk

Rescue Remedy www.bachshop.com

Revitol www.thecellulitereport.com or www.beautyok.co.uk

Revlon www.revlon.com

Rimmel www.rimmellondon.com

Rollasole pumps www.rollasole.com

Shapewear www.figleaves.com

Silk'N www.silk-n.co.uk

Skin Doctors www.skindoctors.eu

Slendertone www.slendertoneface.com

Space NK www.spacenk.co.uk

Spanx www.themagicknickershop.co.uk

Sugar Strip Ease www.sugarstripease.com

Sunsense www.sunsense.co.uk

Talika www.talika.com

Therapulse www.naturepeel.co.uk

Tua Tre'nd www.tuatrendface.com

Tweezerman www.tweezerman.co.uk

Ultimo bras www.figleaves.com

Ultra www.ilovebeautyproducts.com

Veet www.veet.co.uk

Vexum.sl™ www.cdwow.com

Xen-Tan www.xen-tan.co.uk

YSL available from all large department stores

ZO www.zoskinhealth.com

For advice, and to find a therapist

Breast reduction ops www.nhs.uk/conditions/breast-reduction

Cosmetic acupuncture www.cosmeticacupunctureuk.com

Cosmetic dentistry www.bda.org

Dermatologists consult your GP

General Medical Council www.gmc-uk.org

Hair restoration www.wimpoleclinic.com

Massage therapy www.massagetherapy.co.uk

Moles www.themoleclinic.co.uk

Nutritionists www.findmynutritionist.co.uk

Permanent make-up www.beautyworkslondon.co.uk

Pilates www.pilatesfoundation.com

Plastic surgeons British Association of Aesthetic Plastic Surgeons
www.baaps.org.uk

Power Plates www.powerplate.com

Spas www.spabreak.co.uk

Universal contour wraps www.universalcontourwrap.com

Acknowledgements

I'd like to thank all the loyal women (and men!) who have been with me from when Harley Street was just a dream and are still with me now, in this fabulous reality!

I'd also like to thank my editors Liz Gough and Lorraine Green at Pan Macmillan for welcoming me into the family.

Special thanks goes to Daniel Galvin and Cristiano for servicing my hair! Jan Marini for inspiring me with her wonderful insight into skincare. Lifelong friend David Hicks for all his support and extra special thanks to my agent and friend Neil Howarth who always believed in me – we did it!

On a personal note I'd like to say a special thank you to my mother and father and sisters for giving me so much support and encouragement during this amazing journey through life! I am blessed.

Index